How to Be a
Cut Above
Your Competitors

How to Be a
Cut Above
Your Competitors

Insider Secrets for Positioning Your Way
to the Top of the Cosmetic Surgery Market

Nick Dumitru

How to Be a Cut Above Your Competitors
*Insider Secrets for Positioning Your Way to the
Top of the Cosmetic Surgery Market*

Copyright © 2013 by Nick Dumitru

Hardcover: 978-0-9921136-1-2
Paperback: 978-0-9921136-0-5
eBook: 978-0-9921136-4-3

Contents

About This Book   *vii*

Foreword   *ix*

CHAPTER 1 – It's Not Easy Being the Doctor   1

CHAPTER 2 – Understanding the Plastic Surgery Buyer   9

CHAPTER 3 – The 9 Dumbest Things Doctors Do   17

CHAPTER 4 – Conversion   45

CHAPTER 5 – Positioning for Success   97

CHAPTER 6 – The Attraction Side of the Formula   111

CHAPTER 7 – Strategy vs. Tactics   117

CHAPTER 8 – Is It an Expense or an Investment?   129

CHAPTER 9 – Marketing Not Only Attracts But Also
            Selects a Customer   133

Bibliography   *143*

About This Book

If your practice isn't as busy as it should be, if your phone isn't ringing enough, or not at all, if you're losing too much business to your competitors, if you get too many tire kickers in your office, if you don't enjoy selling, or if you simply want more—then it will definitely pay to read this book.

This book is not intended to be an elaborate exercise in theory. It's not meant to pump you up with hope while giving you nothing solid to act upon. This book is a practical guide, using real-world strategies and a battle-tested, proven, formula for success—tactics and strategies that I've used to help my clients dominate their respective cities, regardless of the economic climate; the same techniques that propelled single physician practices into multimillion-dollar businesses.

I don't pull punches and I don't waste words. I'm going to get right to the point. I may use some questionable language from time to time, so if you have a sensitive disposition, please stop reading now. If you can handle a little grit and you want to succeed, read on.

Growing a practice is formulaic. It's simple and works every time—provided you have a proven formula. This book is about that (practice growth) formula.

It's my hope that you'll use the enclosed information and take action toward your own success.

Foreword

Plastic surgeons competing in the aesthetic marketplace face a new reality in practice today.

While we are well-trained in the intricacies of plastic surgery, we have not been trained to develop our practice to address the wants of our patients.

As cosmetic surgery has become more mainstream, the business of aesthetic medicine has grown, and so has the competition for patients. We were never taught, however, marketing and sales in medical school.

This is not just another book about marketing. It's about understanding the patient's desires, differentiating oneself in a competitive market, and then delving into all aspects of one's business practices, not simply Internet marketing but across the spectrum from print ads to how the phone is answered by your staff.

When I first brought Nick in to work with my practice, I was doing okay but consultations were on a downward trend and I was spending time with people that needed convincing. Once his marketing machine kicked in, it all changed. My waiting list is five to six months long and I'm seeing the kinds of patients I want to see. My consultations are more about going over patient concerns than trying to convince them that I'm the right surgeon to go with. Many of the patients that "shop" five or six surgeons are gone.

My biggest challenge bringing on a marketing expert was the cost of the investment. As Nick points out, never make the mistake of confusing an expense with an investment. An expense has no yield. An investment returns money on your dollar. If your marketing can return a multiple of what you invest, it is in your best interest to invest in that marketing, and to invest heavily.

And so it has been with my practice.

Dr. Jerome Edelstein, MD, FRCSC
Plastic Surgeon
Toronto, Ontario, Canada

CHAPTER 1

It's Not Easy Being the Doctor

The cosmetic surgery business is brutally competitive and it's getting worse every day. The market is commoditized and consumers are making choices based on price. Your profit margins are being squeezed and you make less than you used to make even a few short years ago. You're working just as hard but are getting a diminishing return on your time and effort.

When people see you for consultations, too many of them seem to just be kicking the tires or shopping around. Their final decision often comes down to price. They try to haggle and see if they can get your services at a lower rate. Why is it, you wonder, that some of your colleagues seem to be getting away with charging more? What is it that allows them to ask a premium while your prospects generally seem to want to go for the lowest price? Are they better than you? You *know* they're not.

You have a pair of skilled hands—hands that can change people's appearance and their lives. You know you're good at what you do. Your practice isn't doing badly, but it isn't at the level you want it to be, or you know it should, and could, be.

When you're sitting at your computer and Google your competition, you see them doing well online. You look at photos of their clinics and wonder how they can justify the opulence.

How can they pay for their numerous staff and for all the latest equipment? Sure, you *could* pay for it but it would make no sense to your accountant. It would take years to recover the expense, and by that time, the next new gadget would make your machine obsolete. You're not in business to be a slave to your suppliers.

You go out to dinner with your wife, on one of the few nights you didn't work late at the office or are too tired to enjoy yourself. As you park your car, you notice one of your colleagues pulling up as well. (You call him a colleague but deep down you know he's nothing more than a competitor.) He's the guy treating the patients that should have gone with you. He steps out of his exotic car and you give him a fake smile and nod. If your practice was doing as well as his, you guys might even be friends. But it's not. And you can't stand it. His skills are nothing special, there's no doubt about that. When he messes up, his patients come to you. They cry about what he did to them. You shake your head, knowing how little he deserves his spectacular success. Can people not tell that you're better; don't your results speak for themselves?

This encounter also gives you time to ponder. Why is it that you go out and enjoy yourself so seldom these days? And what about the kids—it feels like you can't find nearly enough time to spend with them. You're always working, and sometimes you wonder if it's really worth the sacrifice.

You want to have what he has. You want his kind of success. No, you *DESERVE* it. You're the better surgeon, the better injector, the better doctor overall. You *KNOW* you should be winning at the plastic surgery business and yet, in a business sense, you still seem to fall short. It's simply not right and you know it.

If only you could get the number of patients he gets. If only you knew how he manages to pull in so much business while the industry is hit by the economic downturn. If only you knew how this whole online marketing thing worked. He must just be lucky. Yeah, that's it. If only you had his luck. If only.

The truth is that luck has nothing to do with it. It's a cop-out but you don't know what to do about it, so you accept it, knowing it's not the truth. Knowing that there has to be a way to do better, to get more patients, to show the world your skill and your superior abilities. You yearn for significance. You *need* to be great. Plastic surgery is what you were meant to do; it's your calling and that's why you paid your dues in medical school. You spent long nights studying and gave up so much, hoping to be so much more.

> *"Resentment is like taking poison and*
> *hoping the other person dies."*
> **—Augustine of Hippo**

Being less successful than you want to be isn't your fault. You're not dumb. You didn't get where you are because you're stupid. But they didn't teach you marketing and sales in medical school and you **have** been fed a load of nonsense for a long time. Ever since childhood, you've been told all manner of lies about success. Everyone from your parents to your teachers, cartoons and popular culture have been feeding you the same sort of messages over and over, brainwashing you and putting you on the path to mediocrity. Things like:

"Just work hard and you'll do well."

"If you do good work, people will come to you."

"Good always triumphs over evil."

"Word of mouth is the best form of advertising."

"Sales is a dirty business."

"If you're really that good, you shouldn't have to advertise."

"If you build it, they will come."

BULL!

The reality is that even the best products and services in the world will fail to achieve solid market penetration without proper marketing, positioning, differentiation, and promotion. If billion-dollar companies can and do fail, do you think you can do nothing and expect to succeed? Brainwashing is insidious and you need to break free the moment you finish reading this sentence.

It's Not as Hard as You Think If You Have a Proven Formula

It's not difficult to make very good money in the cosmetic surgery business. I've helped build seven- and eight-figure businesses. The main thing I learned and noticed is that practice number two was easier than number one, and number three was even easier to grow than the previous ones, and so it goes. Distilling what I've done into a repeatable formula makes the process predictable and reliable.

This book is about that formula, something I have never shared with anyone before. Not even our clients knew exactly what we did in order to generate the massive business growth they enjoy. This is the first time I've ever made it public. It outlines the steps we took to add wealth. It goes through the methodology and tactics we used to build successful practices for anyone we took on.

The Practice Growth Formula boils down to this:

$$C(a+d) \times T(ms) \times ORM = GTNP$$

Conversion (appeal plus differentiation) multiplied by Traffic (from multiple sources) multiplied by Online Reputation Management, equals Growth Through New Patients.

It's not as hard as you think but it's not easy by any means. It takes work and, above all else, it takes action. Take the first step by going through this book and understanding why you're not where you want to be. By the time you're done, you'll know exactly what needs to be done. You'll understand why your competitors have an edge and how you can eliminate that advantage. You'll learn how to marginalize them and become the dominant leader in your city. Read every page and read this book to the end.

The Formula is tested and it's proven to work. It works in a bad economy. It works in a saturated market. It works as long as you implement it in its entirety.

My knowledge is not theoretical. It doesn't come from a textbook and it's not parroted corporate speak. I didn't get it by reading some blog about plastic surgery marketing or how to convert sales online. I learned what I know, and what works, by doing: By getting my hands dirty in the trenches. By learning with every dollar spent on ads and with every click on a search engine result. By designing websites and optimizing them to yield massive profits for doctors just like you. Once we got into the mind of our clients' prospective market, we applied our discoveries across all their marketing efforts, from print ads to websites and right down to how the phone is answered. Everything we learned fed the marketing machine and helped the whole system perform stronger.

When I started online, Lycos and Excite were battling it out with Yahoo!, and Google was just a glimmer of an idea. I've been watching and working the Internet for a long time. I would say it's a lifetime in dog years, but the truth is that *Internet years* move a lot faster. During all these years, tactics have changed. Technology has changed. Even where and how we place ads is drastically different. But the one constant has been the psychology and the motivation of the cosmetic buyer. What motivated her over a decade ago is the exact same thing driving her decisions today, and it will be the same thing long after I'm dust. It's that keen understanding of the subtle nuances of the female mind that allows me to do what I do.

I can only do what I do because I understand the buyer's mindset. I know how she thinks and what buttons to push.

If you're struggling to get patients to your practice, you don't have to be. The patients are out there for the taking. The biggest problem I have is getting our clients to manage their own growth. We build a dominant leader in any cosmetic market we enter. I hope that never changes and I have no intention of allowing it to.

As their business grows, I'm not always on the frontlines but I'm still fully involved in all major strategic marketing decisions for our clients.

There are times where I may come across as sexist or insensitive. Nothing could be further from the truth. It's my deep respect for women that has allowed me to gain an intense, deep under-standing of how they think, and what they want when buying cosmetic services. I'm not going to bow down to political correct-ness or start injecting variations of he/she in my sentences. It's more important to me that you understand the concepts clearly. If you don't like me referring to doctors as *he*, then just pretend I put an *s* in front of it. I mean nothing derogatory by it. It's simple efficiency.

The one thing I won't apologize for is calling the patient *she*. In most of the practices I've seen, men comprise less than 15 per-cent of the business. In most plastic surgery practices, the men are barely even statistically significant. Unless you exclusively target male-only products or procedures, women are where the business is. They are, by far, the largest demographic when it comes to cosmetic procedures.

Chapter 2

Understanding the
Plastic Surgery Buyer

During my decade-plus in this business, I've gained a profound insight into the mind of the cosmetic buyer, based on testing and observation of buying behaviour, with, literally, millions of dollars of research data gathered from advertising spend. I didn't go around interviewing consumers and sit there listening to them tell me one thing while they did another. Be very wary of that kind of research. What a human being tells you and what she does can be one hundred percent different.

For example, in a neurological study of behaviour performed by M. Lindstrom (2008), smokers were asked if the grotesque and disturbing images placed on cigarette packages were likely to deter them from smoking. The smokers said that the images would deter them. However, when they were shown the actual images, brain scans revealed that the craving sectors of their brains (nucleus accumbens) lit up. The images were actually stimulating their craving for cigarettes. The smokers associated the images with the immediate gratification they felt from lighting up.

What they said and what actually took place in their minds were diametrically opposed realities.

That's just one of the reasons I'll never conduct a focus group again as long as I live.

During the early part of my career, I also saw how pack behaviour led people to a frenzy of opinions that then had absolutely no correlation to buying data. These days I only look at experiment results and real-world consumer behaviour. You can learn more from split testing a few Pay-Per-Click (PPC) ads than you'll ever learn from talking to thousands of buyers. There is an old sales adage that states "buyers are liars" and I can certainly attest to it.

Pay attention to what your patients are actually doing, not to what they say they're going to do—or even worse, to something some consultant tells you she's going to do based on research he got from interviewing patients. That data is flat out useless. If you want play money, then play around with focus group data. If you want real money, pay attention to what's actually happening in the real world.

Fear and Desire: The Twin Sisters of Your Fate

You've no doubt been told that one of the biggest obstacles to cosmetic surgery and non-invasive cosmetic treatments is fear. BULL!

That sort of information is nothing more than corporate drivel dished out by people with a VP title in some large organization; people that have never sold a single vial of toxin or filler themselves; corporate hacks that put together a focus group and watched a pack of women come together to boldly say that they wouldn't try something because they are "afraid."

I didn't realize how wrong the whole fear angle was until I showed a landing page to a friend of mine who is completely removed from the cosmetic industry. He is so removed, in fact, that he'd have to take a boat for an hour or so to even get on a piece of land which may or may not have access to a plastic surgeon. I couldn't ask for a more objective perspective. For someone as close to the cosmetic industry as I am, I love to take advantage of this kind of untainted observation.

The landing page was for a BOTOX® offer and it was generating leads well for this client. It was targeted at women and had a prominent image of the BOTOX® packaging near the top of the page. The conversation with my friend went like this:

"What do you think of this landing page?"

"What the—? It says 'neurotoxin' right there in that picture at the top of the page and it converts? Are they crazy?"

After I stopped laughing, it became crystal clear to me that fear has absolutely no bearing on the situation, and there is scientific proof to support it, which I'll explain later.

First, let's examine what the landing page said. The line on the packaging he was referring to was *botulinum toxin type A*. A quick Google search for botulinum toxin brings up the Wikipedia page for the subject. The very first paragraph on that page says the following, verbatim:

Botulinum toxin is a protein and neurotoxin produced by the bacterium Clostridium botulinum. It is **the most acutely toxic substance known,** with an estimated human median lethal dose of 1.3–2.1 ng/kg intravenously or intramuscularly and 10–13 ng/kg when inhaled. **Botulinum toxin can cause botulism, a serious and life-threatening illness in humans** and animals. Popularly known by one of its trade names, BOTOX®, it is used for various cosmetic and medical procedures.[1]

"THE MOST ACUTELY TOXIC SUBSTANCE KNOWN."

Keeping that in mind, now realize that Allergan sells roughly $650 million worth of BOTOX® every year for cosmetic use. They produce it in a secret and secure facility because of the danger that it can be used as a biological weapon. Women all over the world are injecting **"the most acutely toxic substance known"** into their bodies to get rid of a few wrinkles.

So ... fear is one of the biggest deterrents to cosmetic services? Really?

The person who undergoes cosmetic surgery has a psychological profile that is not risk-averse. This means that she is not afraid of the potential consequences of her actions. She lives on desire. Desire is what you need to target; offer the risk reassurance as a secondary tool for her to use to fend off her detractors who don't want her to undergo the operation. In the end, she'll do what she wants, but make no mistake about it: Fear is not her primary motivator for or against the procedure.

What the corporate hacks are referring to is the population at large. Corporations are concerned with lines on paper that tell them that they need to broaden the market—that they need more people to use their products and that they need to educate the consumer. Then, they pass that information down to you and make you do part of their dirty work at your expense.

Let me make this easy for you. You're not out to educate the market. You're after the **cosmetic buyer**, not the population at large. Your fastest route to more patients is to attract and convert the patients that are already in the market for your services. Let the large corporations spend the stupid money on mass education and branding campaigns. For you, the smart money is in going after people who are already buying—not in trying to create more of a market for the corporations.

There is a place for fear in marketing cosmetic services but fear is your ally, not your adversary. Fear is something to be treated with care and respect. I call fear and desire the twin sisters because the gentle pull between fear and desire is what works on the psychology of prospects and converts them into your patients. One is seldom present in the mind without the other.

A concern for wrinkles is driven by the fear of getting old, the fear of losing vitality, and the fear of competition in the mating game. It's also brought along by the desire for beauty, control, and sex. The sisters play havoc on a woman's mind and if you know how to use them correctly in your marketing, you'll be seen as someone that understands her, someone who empathises and can deliver on her desires while simultaneously banishing her fears.

Every service you provide has unique advantages and disadvantages, and the psychology of your prospective buyer personas are different and distinct. The sisters say different things in the mind of a thirty-two-year-old versus a fifty-five-year-old. They hold different conversations in the head of a divorced mother than they do in the head of a single and childless career woman looking to advance in her profession.

You need to first identify whom you're speaking with, then start talking in a tone and using words that she *wants* to hear and that resonate. Only then will you be heard and, more importantly, listened to.

The Message to Market Match

When looking at buyer psychology, you need to understand a few fundamental principles:

1.   **Every service you have is purchased by at least one distinct buyer persona, often up to four.**

2.   **Every buyer persona needs to be sold in a different way.**

Dermal fillers are a great example of a single product that has distinct buyer personas.

Fillers are used to non-surgically enhance facial features, augment the lips, reduce wrinkles, and modify the nose, cheeks, or jawline. Although it's one product, it has several distinctly different uses, each of which tends to attract a different type of buyer.

Lip augmentation: The woman coming in for lip augmentation is typically younger and actively in the market for a mate. Or, if she has a mate, she is looking to build her confidence level.

Wrinkles: The woman concerned with wrinkles is typically older and is disturbed by the visible signs of aging. Her concerns have nothing to do with being a sexpot for the sake of it. She's mostly looking to regain something she's lost. Her motivation can be completely different from that of the younger patient.

Modification of other facial features: The woman who is interested in modifying other facial features can vary in age, and her concern is mostly eliminating something she sees as a "problem" feature, something that may have been bothering her for most of her life. Dermal fillers may even be perceived as a preliminary solution, before she proceeds with surgery to achieve permanent results.

Psychological traits may be shared amongst the three. However, there still exist three distinct personas, each of which responds to specific language and other content based on what she cares about and what resonates with her fears and desires. This is not only the case when you're talking to her during a consultation but also when she is reading your written education and/or marketing materials.

So much content put out by plastic surgeons is generic and all-encompassing. Doctors think that if they cast a large enough net, they'll catch a whale. But the market is not comprised of whales. It's comprised of millions and millions of minnows: tiny decisions that a woman has to make before she says *yes* to you. Most fall through the net because the language doesn't speak to her directly.

Identify your buyer and speak only to her in your marketing. Don't try to use a net when a hook is the right, and most efficient, tool for the job. Be precise and be accurate.

If you haven't been paying attention to cosmetic buyers as long as I have, the above can seem daunting, and it is. But that doesn't mean that you can get away with not doing it. If you're satisfied with getting less than you could, use the same generic content given to you by your suppliers. If you want to be the market leader, start positioning your services in a way that differentiates you from your competitors.

CHAPTER 3

The 9 Dumbest Things Doctors Do

Nobody Cares About You (Well, Except Maybe Your Mother)

I was sitting in a meeting with a client and a "business consultant" from one of the large medical device companies. Something the "business consultant" said shocked me and made it very clear why so many doctors don't get all they want from their practice. This consultant's advice was to change the hyper-responsive website we built for our client to one that showcased the surgeon. He told my client that patients are online looking for the doctor, so it's the doctor who should be highlighted on the homepage and the foundation on which the site should be built.

WRONG!

Your mother may care about you, but everyone else cares about themselves. Even while reading this book, you don't give a rat's ass about me. You don't want to know what I had for breakfast or how I'm feeling today. You care about your practice, your bank account, and the satisfaction you get from dealing with ideal patients. I'd better tell you something useful and applicable to your business or you're putting this book down and moving on to something of interest to YOU. Your patients are no different.

Your prospective patient isn't on your website to learn about you, no matter who shows up and tells you otherwise—at least not initially. She's there for her own needs. She first wants to know if you can do what she wants you to do. Then, if you're any good at it, she looks for confirmation of your abilities, affirmation of your claims, and proof for herself and other people in her life.

Putting your big face on the homepage addresses absolutely none of her concerns. There is a place and a time for your own positioning and for your photo, and it's not the top of the home page.

My advice isn't based on some unfounded conjecture on my part. It's not based on focus groups or spending ten minutes in the waiting room of some plastic surgery office. It's not based on something some corporate hack told me to tell you so I can make an ego play and try to cozy up to you.

My advice is based on scientifically observing 30,000 to 500,000 visitors a month on websites for over fifteen years. It's based on listening to 1,000-plus hours of recorded incoming calls to cosmetic practices. It's based on training frontline staff to handle incoming calls and helping our clients grow to multimillion-dollar practices. It's real-world knowledge from being down in the trenches and helping surgeons win at the plastic-surgery-practice game. Heed it and you'll win, too. Ignore it and you can comfort yourself with your well-stroked ego. I'm interested in helping you make more money, not in making you feel big. I'll leave that job to your mother because she's the one who cares about you and your sensitive disposition.

Go to your computer. Look at your home page. What is it telling prospective patients about what you can do for them? If this were a blind date, would you be screaming and boasting about how great you are?

If your site is not one hundred percent focused on patient needs, wants, and desires, you need to rethink your website and fire your web design company.

MISTAKE #1
DOING IT ON YOUR OWN

"Time is the scarcest resource, and
unless it is managed, nothing else can be managed."
— Peter Drucker

If You're Doing It All Yourself, You've Already Lost

This is not a time management book, so I'm not going to pretend to teach you about managing your time. However, time is the omnipresent commodity in which we all trade—and nothing could be truer in business and in your practice. From the time you wake up every morning, you have choices to make. You need to decide what you're going to do that day to further your success before your time runs out. If you think you can do it alone, you're probably wrong.

As you read this, keep one thing firmly in mind: **Activity does NOT equal progress.**

THE ROLLER-COASTER EFFECT

When you resolve to do things yourself, you get sucked into the roller-coaster effect. I've observed this phenomenon in business and in online marketing. The physician thinks he can do things on his own and puts all his effort and energy into trying to get business. He has a modicum of success and business starts to go up. It's exciting. It exhilarates him, but now he has to start servicing the clients obtained from his efforts. This is the tip of the first rise of the roller coaster, when you feel the most excitement and anticipation at what's happening. But it's also the start of the scary drop down, the realization that you're no longer in control and gravity is about to have its way with you.

He performs the surgeries but has no time to focus on the marketing. Things slip. Content is no longer created. Business starts to fall. He sees the bottom and decides to focus on marketing again because business is slowing down. The roller coaster goes back up. Then down again. Then up. Then the fatigue causes him to make mistakes so he's sent for a loop. He recovers and goes back up.

The story can continue for months or years but the end result is always the same: The ride comes to an end. The surgeon is spent and the business is just a fraction of what it could have been.

Your goal is not to be on a roller coaster. You need to get off the ride and get serious about your own success. You're after a rocket-like trajectory which puts you on a path to getting everything you want out of life. Why limit yourself to the roller-coaster ride of the do-it-yourselfer when the universe can be yours?

Successful organizations are built by people working together toward a common goal. No major surviving corporation was started by one person alone. They were all started by at least two individuals. Think Steve Jobs and Steve Wozniak of Apple; Bill Gates and Paul Allen of Microsoft; or closer to home, Gavin S. Herbert and Stanley Bly of Allergan, or the Johnson brothers of Johnson & Johnson.

Still think you can do it all alone? You're still wrong. You only have twenty-four hours in a day. By definition, you cannot scale yourself. Put your ego aside and identify your weaknesses. Then, find key people to make up for your shortcomings, allowing you to focus on what you do best: plastic surgery.

Doing it alone sounds good in movies and fairy tales, but that kind of thinking has no place in a successful practice.

In my experience, I've observed different physician personalities. A few got it right, but most got it horribly wrong. Let's examine a few of the typical personas I've encountered, into which you may or may not fall partially or wholly.

The important thing is not just recognizing where you are; it's recognizing where you should be and then taking the steps to get there. Focus on the future, because you can't change the past and there is no point in worrying about it.

THE BUMBLER

I've seen this personality come in two varieties: either incredibly intelligent or incredibly stupid. The dumb ones don't last long or get very far, so I won't waste time on them. Instead, I'll tackle the intelligent Bumbler. This individual is often very good at what he does and is highly intelligent. So much so, in fact, that it leads him to a couple of key limiting beliefs:

1. "Nobody can do things as well as I can, so I should do it myself."

2. "I'm so smart. I can do that. Why spend the money hiring someone to do it?"

These are beliefs typically accompanied by self-delusion and what Cambridge researchers identified as *The IKEA Effect*: a human need to overvalue the things we create (Arieli et al., 2011).

The Bumbler is smart so he enjoys a modicum of success. He has patients from the sheer volume of activity and effort he puts in, but he never sees any real wealth. His business traps him and pulls him down into a stressful situation. He ends up working for his business instead of making it work for him. In effect, he just creates a well-paying job for himself. It's not scalable and is highly time-consuming.

He loves the feeling of being needed and being the centre of his business. But he doesn't realize that being the centre also means he can never break out. His self-delusion lets him believe that he's achieving great things and that his work is good and meaningful. Unfortunately, his marketing materials and positioning are often mediocre because the writing, design and content he produces is only great in his own mind. It doesn't resonate with the market. He'll keep bumbling along until he wakes up and makes a change, which is rare, or until it's time to retire, which is most often the case.

With retirement, he won't have a business to sell. As he, the centre, leaves, the spokes come undone and the practice falls apart, quietly.

These situations are responsible for the sad calls that come in to my clients' offices from patients with doctors who have retired or passed away, as they scramble to find another doctor to perform more of the surgeries they want.

Wouldn't it have been great if he nurtured a junior well ahead of time to continue his legacy and profitability? The Bumbler is just building his ego and working a job. He has no business to stand on and nothing will carry on after it's time for him to go. While he may enjoy some of the financial trappings that come from his activity, he never sees any truly meaningful success. The Bumbler fooled himself into thinking he has a practice instead of a job.

THE CHEAPSKATE

This penny-pinching tightwad is constantly concerned with how much things cost, how much he's paying out, how much work his suppliers are going to do for the money. His personality can range from timid to arrogant. To him, activity often equals progress. He operates on several limiting beliefs.

1. "Buying things is bad."

2. "People are out to rip me off."

3. "You can't fool me. I'm smarter than you."

4. "You need my money so kiss my ass first."

This small man (figuratively) can't see the forest for the trees. He lets his competitors take market share because he's too cheap to invest in his own business. He may have spent money with a bad marketing company in the past and because they got it wrong, he thinks he's been there and knows everything. He won't "waste" money on hiring anyone again. He'll just buy the cheapest service he can find because he was advised to get online by some session he attended at an ASPS meeting.

Because of his limiting beliefs, the Cheapskate doesn't invest in his own success. He stays in the same place most of his career. He doesn't make waves. He doesn't expand his business. When it comes time for him to retire, he'll have the money he scrimped and saved. That could be a lot, but it will have been only a fraction of his potential. His kids will also get a fraction of the inheritance he could have left them, and his practice dies the day he retires. His patients have nowhere to turn because he left nobody in charge as a result of his shortsightedness and greed. You cannot hold abundance with a tight fist. Your hands need to be open and giving if you want them to have room to receive.

THE INCOMPETENTLY SUCCESSFUL

The Incompetently Successful personality learned how to promote his business to a relatively successful level. Unfortunately, that's all he learned. The work performed at his practice is typically of low quality with high patient dissatisfaction and poor retention. He survives on the back of his marketing and not much else.

This is the kind of client I refuse to work with for many reasons, mostly because I refuse to grow a shit show.

Once I learned how much power there is in marketing and how many people it can impact, I started being very selective and very careful with whom I help grow. I'm not a big fan of scaling up a headache.

Incompetently Successful surgeons tend to suffer from an exaggerated ego, which comes as a result of the marketing success they've had. They're typically very good at spouting off marketing concepts they barely understand, while at the same time having no idea how to scale and manage their enterprise. This style of practice usually grows to a certain size and then starts to quickly contract. Because the owner only has a rudimentary understanding of marketing and does a lot of it himself, he tends to lose sight of service delivery and his human resources. The end result is either bankruptcy or rapid contraction. This cycle of growth and contraction can go on for several years but ultimately ends badly.

THE CEO SURGEON

The CEO Surgeon is truly a pleasure to work with. He's the type of person that knows his limitations and knows that the path to success is paved with people who can make up for his shortfalls. He knows to put the right people in place to support his expansion and rewards them accordingly. He may have spent the first part of his career being the Cheapskate or the Bumbler, but he's changed and broken free. He opened his mind to possibilities and "grew a pair" when he decided to strategically invest in, and grow, his practice.

This surgeon doesn't try to understand marketing in general, along with search engines and social media, because they're not his core competencies, nor should they be. He focuses his attention on his own strengths and money-generating activities. He's confident but knows when to put ego aside in areas that aren't his core strength and hires experts to do those jobs.

While he's good with his money and monitors expenses, he knows how to differentiate between an expense and an investment.

The CEO Surgeon is what you should aspire to be.

Action Step

Here is an exercise I sometimes get my clients to perform. It helps focus their attention on what they should be doing and identifies what not to do.

Step 1: Keep a diary of your daily activities. Be rigorous and disciplined about it. If you have a weekly routine, keep it for a week. If your routine varies, keep it for a whole month, or as long as you need to establish a reasonably solid pattern of activities.

Step 2: Identify and grade all the activities you perform in your business. Separate them by Competence Level, Enjoyment, and Contribution to your bottom line.

Give anything that you're exceptionally good at/gifted at, you enjoy doing, and makes you money an 'A' rating.

Give anything that you're exceptionally good at and contributes to the bottom line but is not enjoyable a 'B' rating. Many surgeons I've met rate injectable fillers and BOTOX® as such.

Give anything you're not exceptionally good at but may enjoy or not enjoy doing a 'C' rating.

Your goal is now to try and focus nearly a hundred percent of your time and energy on 'A'-rated activities. If you want to scale, you need to find people to take over the 'B'-rated activities. Immediately find someone to take on all the 'C'-level activities.

In this exercise, I'm obviously referring to business activities, and there may be a few things you can't let someone else take over. For example, you may have to stay on as the medical director whether you enjoy it or not (at least until your practice grows to a self-sustaining size, after which you will have additional options open to you).

MISTAKE #2
EQUATING ACTIVITY WITH PROGRESS

I see this over and over. It's how most marketing, consulting, SEO, and design companies sell their services. They give the physician a set of activities that are going to be performed. It can range from everything from redesigning their website and posting on Facebook once or twice a day to the numbers of links they'll build for them weekly. It's usually presented as a nice mind map or large list of activities. The doctor feels good because he gets to see all the stuff he's going to get people to do in exchange for his cash. He feels great because he knows that people are "working" for the money.

Activity DOES NOT Equal Progress

If you're paying attention to how much your staff or contractors are doing, you're paying attention to the wrong metrics. It's not about the level of activity, it's about results. If what you're doing doesn't rank your site higher in search engines and doesn't convert more prospects to paying patients, which ultimately puts more money in your bank account, they're doing the wrong things.

Running around in a circle doesn't mean you're taking a single step forward. All your efforts and metrics should be designed to move your business forward, not make you feel like someone else is doing something. Thinking you're getting value for your money doesn't mean you actually are. It just means you were well-sold and well-managed.

When I walk into most practices and evaluate their efforts, it always reminds me of my time as a young boy. When I was growing up, I'd watch my grandparents kill a chicken for dinner. They would grab a chicken from the yard and quickly sever the head off with a knife. The chicken would then thrash around the yard for what seemed like 30 minutes to me at the time, until it exhausted all its blood and effort. It was then ready for plucking and cooking.

Most practices are no different. They stick their neck out unwittingly and put their fate in the hands of a marketing amateur with a good portfolio, featuring other chickens he's plucked.

These practices soon find themselves expending tremendous effort in accomplishing no meaningful action. Their thrashing around doesn't save their failing practice. They put their faith in the hands of a butcher. It pains me to see so many in my profession with so little knowledge and understanding of what marketing and the Internet are about. Computers have leveled the playing field, but they've also lowered the bar.

Whatever you're doing, stop. Take a look at your activity and ask yourself if it has made a *meaningful* difference in your business—and I'm not talking about modest growth you can expect in most practices over time. I use the word "meaningful" very deliberately. Are your efforts having a life-changing, transforming effect on your practice? Are they propelling you to the head of the industry in your city? If the answer is *no*, you're probably equating activity with progress. You need to stop and focus on the things that move you **forward**.

"It is an immutable law in business that words are words, explanations are explanations, promises are promises —but only performance is reality."
—Harold S. Geneen

MISTAKE #3
START-STOP MARKETING

I don't even need to be working with a practice to know if they're suffering from this. All I have to do is look at their website and social media.

The signs are all over the place: You start a blog. You're excited about it because some moron told you it's the way to rank your site and engage your audience. But it isn't working for you. Your site doesn't rank better. People are not reading the blog. After a month or two, you decide the expense isn't worth it and you stop.

Next, you attend a session at one of the annual meetings where another supposed expert has you absolutely convinced that if you're not on Facebook and Twitter, you're losing out. You tell your staff to quickly open a Facebook account and set up a page, which you then start to spam with your own activities, thinking that people actually give a rat's ass about what you're doing. You're wrong again. It doesn't engage people or help your practice. You relegate it to the backburner and post once a week, or less, just to make it look like you're doing something in social media and have that base covered in your mind. Yet, it does next to nothing in growing your practice. You just assume it's a dead end.

The net result from all these efforts is that what you were told doesn't work. It couldn't be your incompetence in the medium, could it? Of course it's not you, it can't be! Your competitors are just lucky. Your prospective clients don't use Facebook. You think of every excuse under the sun, other than the fact that maybe, just maybe, you're doing it wrong because you were told WHAT to do, but not HOW to do it.

MISTAKE #4
LETTING "EXPERTS" TELL YOU WHAT WORKS INSTEAD OF TESTING IT FOR YOURSELF

We trust experts with our well-being. After all, they know better, right?

This instinct, at its best, drives you to seek competent help for your practice. It drives you to call someone like me who knows exactly where to push and how to aggressively market.

At its worst, it sends you into the hands of companies that look professional with a large client list; the kinds of companies that help you to equate activity with progress; companies with a pretty portfolio and no financial metrics to back up their claims, with no active testing protocols to show you that what they do makes a difference. These companies are typically better at getting your money than they are at growing your practice.

The truth is that your practice doesn't have to rely on any unfounded principles. You went through medical school learning to test and observe. You learned the science and the art of medicine. Marketing is no different. While the artistic component does rely on you hiring an expert, you don't have to rely solely on his opinion. There is only one relevant opinion that matters when it comes to practice growth.

Listen to the Market

The market will tell you if you're doing the right things or the wrong things. The market votes with the only thing that matters to a practice: dollars and cents. If you change your website, the only goal for that site is to drive more patients through your doors and into your waiting room. It's to put people on your operating table and money in your bank.

> *"There is only one boss—the customer.*
> *And he can fire everybody in the company from the chairman on down, simply by spending his money somewhere else."*
> **—Sam Walton**

If you don't have multiple incoming telephone numbers for your different marketing channels, such as your print ads and website, you're operating blind.

If you don't know how your web pages are converting your visitors, you don't know what your site is doing.

If you don't know which PPC ad and landing page combination is more likely to convert the prospect, you're wasting your time and money.

If you don't listen to incoming calls to determine if your staff are saying the right things and booking those precious leads, you're just plain dumb. (Check your local laws before you do this.)

If you're not testing, you, quite literally, don't know what you're doing.

MISTAKE #5
CONFUSING TACTICS WITH MARKETING

By far, one of the biggest mistakes I see doctors make is confusing individual tactics with marketing. I see them jump on all kinds of bandwagons, from search engine optimization to print advertising and social media. They see someone doing something or they attend a seminar at a convention and think that the one tactic they heard about will make *the* difference to their practice.

If you think doing more of what doesn't work will get you more business, you really needed to read this book. If what you're doing now in terms of your positioning, your writing, and your offer isn't working, you can't implement any of it and, reasonably, expect it to work.

I once knew a doctor who thought hiring consulting help cost too much and he could do the search engine optimization (SEO) work himself. He carried a copy of *Search Engine Optimization For Dummies*, and he was definitely a dummy. As of the time of this writing, he has not been able to dominate online, though he's had that book for a few years now.

As we unravel the Practice Growth Formula (more about the formula later), you'll understand why it matters if you rank #1 on Google, but if you don't have your conversion taken care of, you're STILL in trouble.

If you don't understand *why* something isn't working, doing more of what isn't working WON'T get you success. Continuing to do it won't allow you to understand why it's failing. And there is something that is more important, and needs to be taken care of before you should ever consider getting more leads from the web, or anywhere else.

Properly marketing your company means having a plan and then making sure that everything you're doing drives that plan forward. Jumping on the latest bandwagon won't get you where you want to be.

"Don't use the conduct of a fool as a precedent."
—The Talmud

MISTAKE #6
COPYING THE COMPETITION

When you emulate a competitor, the most you can expect to do is 10 to 20 percent better than them—though you're likely doing worse because you're always behind and, most likely, not doing anything better. People don't want to do business with the "also-ran." They want to do business with the leader. They *want* to feel special and they *want* to feel like they're getting the best. When you copy, you're not the best. You're not an innovator and, to put it in layman's terms, you're just not cool enough.

As a copycat, you're doing nothing more than following. You'll never be able to dominate and you risk being put out of business by the next innovation.

The iPhone didn't gain large market share because it was just another phone; it led the smartphone category because it changed things. It did something nothing else could do. It brought together your phone, Internet, music, and photos at a time when most phones could barely make a clear call. It empowered the user and gave her EXACTLY what she wanted, even though she didn't know she wanted it up to that point. It focused on the psychology of the user and her needs and desires and wrapped them around a phone because that's what people understood it as. It was a killer product marketed in the right way, in a way that it could be understood, accepted and, most importantly, desired.

If you want to lead, you have to innovate. However, while you should never lose sight of your competition, don't confuse having to watch them with having to copy them. When they zig, you need to zag—and zag strategically (more about that later).

> *"Whenever you find yourself on the side of the majority,*
> *it is time to pause and reflect."*
> **—Mark Twain**

MISTAKE #7
COMPETING ON PRICE BECAUSE
YOU HAVE NO POSITION

"I have to lower my fee because my competitor is charging less."

That's the rallying cry of the surgeon who doesn't understand buying habits and buyer psychology.

A cosmetic patient makes a buying decision very carefully. The final decision is based on many factors, but the only time price becomes a factor is when you're viewed as a commodity.

To understand commoditization, you have to understand what that means to a cosmetic practice. A *commodity* is defined as follows: a good for which there is demand, but which is supplied without qualitative differentiation across a market.

Without qualitative differentiation across a market. What is the consumer left with when you strip away all aspects of quality and service? She's left with price. Price, therefore, is the only factor left on which she can make a buying decision. So, the problem is not your price—it's that you've allowed the market to strip you of all qualitative aspects on which a consumer can plant her opinion and justify doing business with you.

Neurotoxins are a great example of a cosmetic commodity. These days, everyone from dentists to nurses inject toxins. The large corporations that produce them don't care if YOU go out of business because the demand is there and they make the same amount of money if you charge $15 a unit or $5 a unit. Their margin is fixed. In fact, because of the rewards and discount programs they offer as incentives to do volume, they actually make more if you sell less and they spread the sales around multiple physicians. Their profit is higher and the demand in the market is no better or worse, no matter how many plastic surgeons and dermatologists go out of business.

The story I always tell doctors in order to illustrate this concept is the "Peach Story." If you walk into a supermarket and see a display of locally grown peaches, how do you decide among them? They're all grown on local farms. They're all beautiful and fragrant. The only difference is the price: one is $3.99 per pound, another is $1.99 per pound, and yet another is $0.99 per pound. Most people would simply go on price. Why pay more for the same thing right?

Wrong.

The problem isn't the price; it's that each of the farms and the merchandiser at the store did a poor job in differentiating the product.

Let's look at the same set of peaches. The only difference now is a set of small signs above each one. The $3.99 peaches are local and organic from heirloom groves, which are proven to have a 20 percent higher nutritional content for the same calories. The second set of peaches are conventional, from a local cooperative farm collective that supports your daughter's soccer team every year. The last set are GMO peaches grown with the use of pesticides and chemical fertilizers in an attempt to reduce production costs.

We now have three sets of peaches that were positioned

deliberately to match a set of radically different buying criteria. You can now make a decision based on your personal belief system.

If money is not a huge factor for you, you're health conscious, and you care for the environment, you'll pay a premium for the organic peaches.

If you feel a strong sense of gratitude for what the cooperative is doing for your child and her sports team, you'll pay a premium for the cooperative peaches.

If you're money conscious and only care about price, you'll pick the GMO peaches.

The point being that if you want to charge a premium, you have to differentiate your product so it resonates with the consumer you want to attract. If you want problem patients that are just going to haggle you down on price, by all means, put out rock bottom prices. If you want high quality patients that pay a premium, find out what resonates with them and add it to your positioning.

Think about it. What kind of car do you drive? Was it the cheapest on the market? Why isn't every car on the street the cheapest car available? People don't buy on price unless they have no other discernible choice.

It's your solitary duty to ensure that you're not a commodity, and to give your buyer justification to pay you more for surgery or injectables. Then, when she comes into your office, you have to deliver on your promises. That's how you stop complaining about price and start cashing in. Be advantageously different and earn the business.

MISTAKE #8
CHANGING FOR THE SAKE OF CHANGE

One of my clients had a simple strategy for his advertising. He just changed things all the time. He rarely ran the same ad twice. There was no overriding strategy other than change. He had no reason for doing it other than a gut instinct that it needed to be done.

His biggest problem was that he didn't test. He didn't have a way to gauge how much business was coming in from which advertising vehicle. He just lumped everything together and hoped for the best. The problem with that kind of thinking is that you're very likely to kill a profitable marketing vehicle instead of an underperforming one. If you're not testing and tracking, you have ZERO idea of what's working and what's not working.

John Wanamaker was a wealthy merchant, considered, by some, to be the father of modern advertising. He's famous for the following saying: "Half the money I spend on advertising is wasted; the trouble is I don't know which half."

In today's day and age of custom and recordable phone numbers, instant advertising testing on Google, split testing software, and more, there is absolutely no reason to operate with the kind of ignorance my past client did. It's unfortunate for him that he didn't listen and change his ways. But I learned long ago that I cannot, and should not, care more about a client's business than they do.

MISTAKE #9
LETTING YOUR STAFF DICTATE YOUR MARKETING, INSTEAD OF THE MARKET

It's tempting to assume that if *you* like something, *everyone* must like it too. I see far too many cosmetic surgeons that fall into this line of thinking. You might be guilty of the same. You add products and services because you, your staff, or your wife likes them. You oversee the creation of a web page and assume it's great simply because you had a hand in it. You set your office hours to match your schedule and keep these hours, giving no thought to the needs of your prospective clients.

The fact of the matter is that there is only one opinion that matters to a practice: the opinion of the patient. And by that, I don't mean that you should run surveys and add every suggestion that comes out of one of them. I mean that you need to focus your practice around the needs, wants, fears, and desires of the market.

Business is simple. The market will always tell you if you're doing the right things or the wrong things.

Through careful and controlled testing, you can easily find out if you're doing the right things to grow your business. In fact, you never have to guess at buying new equipment or adding a service if you're willing to put a little bit of money towards careful testing (e.g., by running some Pay-Per-Click campaigns).

Let's assume a rep comes to you with the latest and greatest piece of technology that she swears up and down is in high demand. You're not sure what to do because it's a huge financial investment and reps often exaggerate consumer demand. A controlled test will safely and easily produce data indicating the equipment's worth, or lack thereof.

You can run an ad targeting the brand name of the service or device, which will immediately tell you what the consumer demand is for that exact machine in your area. Send those ads to a landing page promoting a special introductory offer for the treatment to anyone that fills in a form.

This will let you gauge the number of potential serious buyers. Even if you don't buy the equipment, you now have a list of potential patients you can make an alternate offer to. You'll, of course, have to be honest on the page and tell people that the offer is under consideration, and you have to comply with all your local disclosure laws (I'm not a lawyer, so ask yours about these laws). However, you will now know what the right decision is based on what the market tells you.

Easy!

I had a client that let his twenty-something-year-old office manager decide what treatments and services to offer, without any consideration for the market. If she liked it, it was often added. He refused to listen to reason when I discussed this with him because of the strong bond of trust she had built with him over the years. The result was a constant waste of profits on purchasing bandwagon equipment for treatments that were little more than passing fads. They were sometimes profitable over the long run, but it left little on the table for marketing and business stability.

When he hit hard times due to legal fees, he had to cut back on a lot of his marketing. His business stopped growing and started contracting. That was, of course, after I stopped working with him. Had he paid more attention to the market and less attention to the whims of his staff, he would have been able to weather any financial storm because the demand for his services would have remained high, thereby avoiding cutting marketing spend.

Another mistake I see in this same vein is office hours. Most medical offices are open during regular business hours. Unfortunately, nine to five is also when most of your clients are at work. With the exception of soccer moms and the independently wealthy, the vast majority of your potential market is at work.

For surgical services, you might be able to get away with keeping those luxurious hours. However, if you want to run a robust injectable and skin treatment business in addition to surgeries, you need to start taking into account when your *market* is available, not when your staff want to go home.

All this really boils down to one simple concept: do what's right for your client and that will end up being what's right for your business. Start using your patient's logic and decision-making path as opposed to your own. It's not about what you do. It's about what you do for *them*.

CHAPTER 4

Conversion

The Practice Growth Formula Revealed

C(a+d) x T(ms) x ORM = GTNP

Conversion (appeal plus differentiation) multiplied by Traffic (from multiple sources) multiplied by Online Reputation Management, equals Growth Through New Patients.

The Formula starts with conversion.

How You Can Afford to Buy All the Business You'll Ever Need

There is a common misconception among physicians that if they only had more web traffic or were as lucky as their competitors, they could get more patients.

The truth is that, when it comes to online marketing, you can buy all the traffic your site and your practice can possibly handle. All you need is money and knowhow. In spite of popular belief, high traffic and money are not a chicken-and-egg scenario. Your business needs conversion first, not traffic.

Conversion and attraction (traffic) are two sides of the same coin, and to bank that coin you need to have both. However, traffic without conversion is far more useless than conversion without traffic.

By improving your positioning, in a way which greatly helps convert the traffic you're already getting, you instantly make more.

For example, let's say you're spending a very conservative $4,000 each month on PPC ads. Those ads convert your web traffic at the rate of about two clients per month. Your gross profit on a surgery is about $4,000. You're spending $4,000 and getting $8,000 back before expenses—not a great return, but not a loss either. It's a good start and the ads are self-financing. The common logic is to then try paying $8,000 and get $16,000 back. In real life, it doesn't work quite like that, but this is a scenario that all novice online marketers try. You can often throw more at an ad and see diminishing returns because the exposure is broadened and, consequently, the audience is not as tightly targeted as before, so your conversion will drop. That's a formula for bankruptcy. Getting more traffic is not the place for you to start. You need to focus on conversions first, and this is why.

Let's take the same scenario. You spend $4,000 and focus on increasing your on-page conversion rate to the point of getting a mere four clients per month from the same online ads and website. You then tweak the ads and get an additional two clients per month. That's four more clients than you were getting, before you started optimizing your conversion rate, for zero additional cost. Your new site and positioning helps you to also convert one of the referrals that was sent to your site by a previous patient. Now you have five patients you didn't have before. That's an additional $20,000 per month in profit.

You use that newfound capital to buy more online ads, hire a marketing company, and put out a print ad. You use the same conversion principles on those efforts and continue to focus on conversion. You increase it further, and soon, you find yourself being able to afford all the online and offline traffic you could ever need, just by focusing on conversion.

If you build it, they won't come, but if you optimize it, more of those who DO come will end up in your office.

Conversion and attraction work together to fuel your business. You're already getting some leads and some online traffic, but before you spend a penny more to attract a new audience, make sure you're ready to convert it. If you're not, you'll be squandering any money you put toward your advertising. Attraction without conversion is not an investment in your business; it's an expense which can bankrupt you.

Positioning for Conversion

Converting a prospective client into an actual patient has everything to do with understanding the psychology behind her buying behaviour. It also has to do with understanding how you compare against the competition.

Set the Buying Criteria and Eliminate the Competition

This is a simple, but powerful, concept that you can use to systematically eliminate the competition. On a large scale, this is what organizations like the American Board of Plastic Surgery® or The Royal College of Physicians and Surgeons of Canada® do for their members as a whole.

The boards give plastic surgeons designations they can use to try and disqualify all other surgeons, in patients' minds, from performing the procedure. These designations are correctly used on many surgeons' sites, with "Board-Certified" or "Double Board-Certified" plastered all over them, and that's great. The problem, however, is that if you're board-certified, and so are the other twenty doctors in your city, then do you really stand out? Are you special in any way?

Sure, you've given the patient a possible way to eliminate all the other non-plastic surgeon competition as an option, but you still have your colleagues to deal with. They're the ones actually taking the business away from you when it comes to the big, profitable surgeries.

Setting the buying criteria is an expansion of that concept. Simply put, in all your marketing communications (website, brochure, social media, etc.), you want to frame and communicate what makes a good buying decision for your prospective patient. You have to make sure that your definition excludes all competition from qualifying based on the criteria *you've* set.

I'll use a quick example to illustrate the concept more clearly.

Let's assume that you're in a city with ten doctors, including yourself. You have hospital privileges, but four of the doctors in the city are completely private with no access to a hospital (whether it's an actual advantage or not is irrelevant). You can make it a *perceived* advantage. The idea is that you can now set the buying criteria as requiring hospital privileges to get better results. You start to educate the patient on the benefits of having access to the hospital, as it provides them with all the safety advantages and pool of experienced medical staff it affords her.

Notice that we've now set the first barrier. It didn't eliminate all the doctors but you've started to narrow the field from ten to six. Assuming the patient agrees with your argument and it matches her way of thinking, you've just improved your odds from 1:10 to 1:6. But there's more work to be done.

You do further research and find out that of the six, only two physicians know how to perform a drain-free tummy tuck. Again, you educate the patient on the benefits of a drain-free operation. Your odds are now 1:3 (the two other doctors, and you). Finally, you know that you use a piece of equipment that results in smaller scars that heal faster with a 40 percent less noticeable appearance. You educate the patient on why that's an advantage. All patients want as little scarring as possible, so this is your key differentiator that finishes off your buying criteria.

Congratulations, you've now become the only choice in that patient's mind. A 1:1 ratio is a recipe for success. While the other nine doctors might match the buying criteria in part, you're the only one that's a perfect fit. You've stacked the deck in your favour and guided the patient's thinking to something she can reason is the only sensible and logical conclusion: to go with you.

Setting the buying criteria is powerful because it uses the psychology of the mind without needing any specialized skills, like expert copywriting ability, design prowess, or knowledge of website programming. It disempowers the competition and makes buying a simple matter for the patient. If you don't do anything egregious on the phone or in person at the consultation, the person is there to buy—not to shop for price or ask silly questions in one of the ten consultations she's planning to go to that month. YOU are the only RIGHT choice in town.

Converting on Your Web Pages

Any page on your site needs to do three things.

1. Tell the prospect what they're looking at.
2. Tell the prospect why they need to interact with your page.
3. Give them a reason to take action.

WHAT IS THIS?

That's the first question anyone asks when they land on a web page. It doesn't matter if it's from a paid ad or a Google search result. The very first things they ask are the following:

- What is this?
- What can I do here?
- Why should I do it?

Your site needs to answer those questions immediately. That means no wasted space at the top of the page and no fancy flash banners. Grab the viewer's attention with content SHE cares about.

WHAT'S IN IT FOR ME?

The next thing you need to pay attention to is adding value to the interaction. You need to figure out what it is your prospect wants, and give it to her. Is she there to learn? Is she there to buy? Is she there to figure out how to measure her cup size?

People are selfish creatures. We all want what we want, when we want it. Your site visitor is not there for your reasons. She's there for HER reasons. Test your ads and your content and figure out why she's visiting the page. Make sure you read the section about the Buying Roadmap (further on in this book) and align your content with her reasons for being there. Don't waste a lot of web real estate building up to the meat. Show her what's in it for her right away.

Getting the content value proposition right is one of the key engagement metrics for a page that very few online marketers divulge. The people who are in the know pay attention to the psychology, not the geography, of the page.

WHY SHOULD I DO IT NOW?

Just because someone is reading your web page doesn't mean they're going to do anything. Every page has multiple conversion steps. There is an internal process your patients go through before they decide to contact you. Most people will tell you to put a "call to action" on the page, to make sure your phone number is there and make sure they can contact you.

DUH! Obviously, having contact information is the bare minimum any site should have.

But let's delve deeper. You need to examine the page and figure out what the patient should be doing next, what she's likely to do and why she should do it. If you put up a PPC ad and drive traffic to an injectable offer, you need to give her a reason to sign up for that offer. If you send her to a page outlining your book, you need to give her a reason to order a copy, or a reason why you should read it.

Enticing someone to do something can take many forms. You can have a limited time offer, which implies scarcity in order to motivate her to take action now. You can give her incentives for taking action, or build up such an overwhelming value proposition that she'd be absolutely crazy not to take it. Whatever you do, make sure you do something. If she has no reason to act, she won't. Just placing a "call to action" button on the page simply doesn't cut it.

Should You Create a Company, Not a Doctor's Office, to Increase Conversion?

Countless books have been written on branding, so if you want to become a branding expert, feel free to read one of those. I'm not here to preach about your brand. I'm here to tell you how easy it is to get branding wrong.

Branding is simply an extension of marketing and positioning. The mistake 99.9 percent of physicians make is thinking that they need to "brand" before they set up an effective position and internal marketing systems. You've probably attended more than one plastic surgery conference with sessions on branding, and how important your brand is and how much you need to brand.

DRIVEL! All of it!

Your brand is simply an extension of your position in the prospect's mind. You should NEVER start with a brand. You have to start with positioning and differentiation. First, set yourself apart and decide where you fit in the prospect's mind and how you'll stand out from your competition.

"Is it better to have a branded business or is it better to open up a doctor's office?"

There is no right or wrong answer to this question. Dr. Smith Plastic Surgeon doesn't have the same resonance or brand value as Smith Plastic Surgery Institute. But the reality is that anyone telling you to position yourself as a business instead of a doctor's office, without examining the competitive landscape, is full of it.

The only thing that matters is how you're positioned against your competitors and how the market is buying. If you study the market and it's full of multi-location medi spas running several surgeons, you can effectively position yourself against them by being the practice that has the personal touch. The one where the patient is more than a number in a computer, and where she will get the personal attention that leads to great and lasting results.

If you're surrounded by other surgeons, and this would be the case in most cities, then you'll do well to break out and become the respected brand. Position yourself to have more money for the latest equipment or better training for your staff as a result of your size. Bind people to your brand and put all the other doctors in one basket, making it easy for the patient to reject them as a whole.

Once you have market dominance, you can start to carefully reposition yourself to combat any changes in the market, buyout competitors, or expand in a strategic manner.

The important thing is to win first and expand second. You can't advance the war if you're constantly losing the battles. Make the right moves, win the right battles, and a brand will emerge over time. Try to build a brand without positioning and you'll squander large amounts of money on ineffective advertising and promotional efforts.

When you recognize your position, you have knowledge of what patients are buying. When you have knowledge, you have power—power you can use to systematically dismantle the competition, winning a war they may not even realize they're fighting. While they pay attention to their website and their advertising, you'll pay attention to the patients' mind and psychology, because that's the only battleground that matters.

Design vs. Content

You're in the business of looking good. If anyone tells you that marketing is not about looking good, they haven't worked in this industry. However, a more correct statement would be that marketing is not JUST about looking good.

Selling and converting web traffic is about trust, credibility, and value. Design is an emotive medium. It's the fastest way to give someone the "right" feeling without them reading a single word on your site. Design is a complex subject and beyond the scope of this book but I'll give you a few tips.

1. Don't obsess over looks.

Once your design meets the bare minimum of professionalism, it's time to move on and focus on the content and the psychology.

Imagine it as a business meeting. Three guys from different companies show up in suits to sell you on a new laser machine. They're all dressed relatively well, clean-cut and impeccably groomed. Do you check to see which one has the Armani suit and gold cufflinks? Most likely not. The only thing that matters at that point is what comes out of their mouths regarding things that you care about, like payment terms, if it actually works, support, and how much money you're going to make with their laser.

If, however, one of them came in dishevelled, that would be a different story. You may not trust him or be comfortable doing business with him. Therefore, get the look to the point that it does the job, then move on because it's not all about the look.

2. Don't waste people's time, and don't create a distraction.

Fancy flashing banners and long graphics with a spinning logo may get you lots of oohs and aahs from your friends but they won't impress your prospect. Always remember that the medium should never get in the way of the message. And, unless you're selling web design, it should never become the message. Your prospective patient may have visited three to five other plastic surgery websites before landing on yours. She may have a list of five others to check out. If you waste her time, she'll exercise her right to click the back button and disappear forever.

3. Get the message right.

If you got the look right and you were able to engage your prospect, the only thing left that matters is getting the message to resonate with her. From this point on, it's all about the psychology and the Buying Roadmap. Skip the self-aggrandizing language and focus on what she's thinking. Get into the conversation in her head and begin a discussion. That is the most important, most time-consuming, but also the most rewarding thing to do. Get it right and you'll build the practice of your dreams.

"Examine the contents, not the bottle."
—The Talmud

Understanding the Buying Roadmap

Most websites and general marketing is targeted at the "now" buyer: the patient who's been around, learned everything, and is ready to book her surgery. You've probably been advised by countless people to put easy-to-access booking forms all over your site, to make sure that people can call and email you at the drop of a hat.

While that is one type of your prospective buyers, a successful and lasting lead generation funnel cannot be built on trying to target the "now" buyer exclusively. That kind of tactic is too vulnerable to market volatility. In an up economy, that's easily masked by the general buying frenzy associated with perceived abundance. It's easy to think your marketing is (doing) great but it may not be anything special. You're just riding the good times. But like all good times, they come to an end. And that's when you know if you did things right or wrong.

A bad market will turn the "now" buyer into the "later" buyer. Purchases are put off and sales quickly dwindle. A bad economy is great for capturing market share if you've been paying attention to the Buying Roadmap. But it's awful if you're relying on economic trends.

The first thing that you have to understand is that the economy should have little to no impact on your success. I've helped clients grow to being the market leaders and dominating their geographic areas in the middle of a global recession. It made absolutely no difference to their rate of success because I didn't allow them to curl up into a little ball and suck their thumb in the corner complaining about the economy.

The fact of the matter is that no market completely contracts to zero. The market is like the ebb and flow of the ocean. There is high tide and there is low tide. The high tide floats all boats, and a complete idiot can float a business under those circumstances. But it's the skilled sailor that knows how to move out with the tide at the right time and keep his boat on the water.

When the market shifts, you need to go where the market

goes. Leave your competitors while you enjoy the benefits of moving with the wave.

If you build a robust lead funnel, you'll be able to take crucial market share away from your competitors during a down economy. In fact, it can give you a distinct advantage because they'll be low on cash and it will push the competition out of business. Their ineffective and reaction-style marketing will see them in financial distress very quickly while you make up for the economic slump by taking patients that would have otherwise gone to your competitors. Even when there is a 10 percent, 25 percent, or even 50 percent drop in overall patients, you can easily make that up by simply grabbing the missing patients from your competition's share of the market.

All of that starts with understanding and respecting your patient's Buying Roadmap.

The Buying Roadmap is comprised of multiple points along a timeline that can extend as far out as over a decade for some procedures, such as breast augmentation.

For the purpose of this book and for the sake of growing your business as quickly as possible, we're going to focus on a twelve-month Buying Roadmap, comprised of an infinite number of patient interaction points that we'll examine in easily understandable chunks. As you understand the different phases, you can begin to craft the content and marketing channels to bring patients into your buying funnel from all the points along the way.

The Buying Roadmap is a process of decision making that ends after the procedure is completed.

The 10 Points Along the Buying Roadmap

1. Insecurity
2. Interest
3. Desire
4. Education
5. Affirmation
6. Determination
7. Action
8. Defence of Choice
9. Commitment
10. Justification of Choice

The 10 Points, in Detail

1. Insecurity: *The root source of all cosmetic surgery buying*

When a patient is looking to have surgery, it's because there is something about herself that is constantly nagging at her. It all stems from some deep-rooted insecurity. If your patient was a hundred percent fully actualized, she'd be growing organic vegetables and chanting in the sunshine while picking flowers to bestow on her fellow human beings to spread joy. But that's not the case.

However small, the desire to make a change stems from a basal level of insecurity that leads to dissatisfaction and a lack of self-confidence, which makes her feel inadequate in her own mind. The intricacies of this process are not relevant, nor is the concept of internal or external influences.

All that's important for you to understand is that the underlying motivation is insecurity, and that you need to carefully, and ethically, engage that part of her psyche.

2. **Interest:** *The beginning of the search for a solution*

At the Interest stage, your prospective patient starts to really focus in on her problem. She may start obsessing over the issue and talking about it with friends or participating in online forums and discussion groups. The focus at this point is the problem and not the solution.

Understanding phase two is important because you'll need to craft your educational content around the problem. Depending on her perceived problem, there could be any number of surgical, injectable, and noninvasive solutions. If you only focus your content around the solution, you could be missing out on this crucial engagement point.

Remember that the Buying Roadmap can be twelve months or longer, which means that your patient could go to your website any number of times before contacting you for a consultation. If you have an ongoing series of touch points with a prospect over the course of a year, you stand to build significant rapport and trust over the length of her buying journey.

It's at this stage that the real business-building process begins. Setting someone on a buying path twelve months out means that you have up to a year to adjust to changing market conditions before you get in trouble. Unlike your colleagues that focus on the "now" buyer and are in survival mode, you have time to adjust and reassess things. You have stable income to invest in advertising, just as it starts to drop in price and your competitors pull out for lack of business. It gives you a significant advantage to gain market share while the industry is contracting, which means that when the inevitable turnaround happens, you'll be poised as the market leader with all the advantages that it brings.

The person in stage two has likely budgeted the money for her procedure. She will spend the next twelve months thinking about, planning, and saving for her operation. You could have a full-blown economic depression and she may still go through with it because she's too invested in the process. This is great news for you and very bad news for your competitors.

It takes a well-thought-out approach and the fortitude to see through a marketing strategy to bring about the stability and prosperity that comes with investing in marketing along the Buying Roadmap and your patients' buying journey.

3. **Desire:** *Where interest turns into a need to do something about it*

In phase three, the journey starts to pick up momentum. It's this momentum that your marketing should focus on accelerating and put the patient on a clear trajectory to a buying decision. And when I talk about a buying decision, I'm referring to a decision to go with you, not with your competitors. It's a subtle difference but an important one to understand.

All too often, surgeons make the mistake of confusing exposure with influence and publicity with results. I once sat with a surgeon and his PR consultant going over his various pieces: videos on local news stations, print articles, and other public relations wins. Well, at least they looked like wins. When I asked how much business it generated, the PR consultant told me it did nothing. I wasn't surprised at all. I have nothing against PR, if done correctly, but simply getting exposure does not influence a patient to do business with YOU.

I explained to this doctor that what he was doing was creating exposure for the procedure and educating the public. He was raising the level of business for everyone in the industry, dissipating his effort across the dozens of other surgeons in the city. He was giving away slices of the pie to everyone and wondering why he was going hungry.

Desire is the point at which you foster and empower the patient to think that she can do something about it. You do this in a way that binds her to you. You engage her in the process and get her on the path to thinking that you're the only option for her. She comes to you believing that what you do is so unique and so advantageous that going to anyone else is just plain wrong.

It's not enough to help someone decide to have liposuction, a nose job, or breast augmentation. You have to make sure that this accelerating momentum points squarely to your front door. The smallest deviation at this point can send her to a competitor who's doing a better job at positioning than you are.

Your prospect is anywhere from one to twelve months out from a final decision. This means that she has a very long distance to travel before talking to you. It's no different from firing a gun. When aiming a gun, a slight deviation at the end of the barrel will result in missing the target by several feet.

The rules for dealing with Desire are the following:

Engage: Engage the patient by joining the conversation already taking place in her head. Use the same wording, tone, and emotion she's expecting to hear so she'll connect, understand, and bond with you.

Align: Align your message to her needs and desires.

Empower: Empower her to make a decision and take the next step.

Design your system to propel your patients to your waiting room at this stage and you'll reap the rewards for decades.

4. Education: *Where you start to become her trusted advisor for life*

As a doctor, you're in a unique position compared to other business people. You already have a great deal of authority. You're already perceived as an advisor. However, you should never take that for granted. You're up against other doctors and you have to be vigilant in gaining and retaining your patient.

Stage four is where you get the opportunity to build rapport and leverage technology to become the go-to source for your prospective patients. At this stage, your patient is ravenous for information. She wants to know what can be done, what her options are, and what the risks are. She wants to know what other people have done, why this is a good idea, and what she's going to tell her family. Most importantly, she wants to know if she'll be happy.

All these things race through her mind until she gets every last question answered. It's at this point that you have to provide all information related to you, your service, and your practice. You want her coming back to your site over and over again, reading, watching, and listening to what you have to say about her solution.

The good news is that you now have the opportunity to build a relationship with her before she spends a single minute with you face to face. You can spend an hour shooting a set of short video clips, which will educate thousands of patients, one viewer at a time. You can invest in content that covers the breadth and depth of her interest while carefully positioning you as her only choice, subtly nudging her along her buying journey until she starts walking to, then running, right through your door to book surgery before she even sees you.

If you think that sounds absurd, it's not. It's what happens to my clients.

The best example I can give of this in day-to-day life is Apple Inc. Go to an Apple store and see how many people go in there to be sold on a product. It's rare, to say the least. People go to the Apple store to BUY a product, not to be SOLD on a product.

"But the aim of marketing is to make selling superfluous. The aim of marketing is to know and understand the customer so well that the product or service fits him and sells itself."
—Peter Drucker

Let me also tell you a story from one of the case studies on our website. When we first took on this client, the frontline staff had to contend with a whole host of objections from patients (potential and current) right down to complaints about the $100 consultation fee. Tire kickers and price shoppers constantly called just to ask about the fees. The situation was causing a lot of frustration and leading to a declining trend in consultations and booked surgeries over a three-year period.

Using the strategies and tactics outlined in this book, we completely repositioned the client and his office and created objection handling points and credentialing scripts.

A little over a year on, the situation completely reversed. Patients now vie for surgical times and book surgery before they even see the doctor. Staff book fifteen-plus surgeries a month in this way. Their biggest challenge now is making sure they fit the person in for the consult and pre-op appointments before the surgery date, which they do expertly.

Use this as a benchmark for your marketing. If you often find yourself selling, something is wrong with your approach.

5. Affirmation: *Where social proof justifies her decision*
Stage five sees your client beginning to justify her

decision to do something about her concern. She may be facing many social stigmas, pressures, and misconceptions about cosmetic procedure. She likely has a lot of fears, everything from paralysis as a result of BOTOX® to not waking up from anesthesia. As a doctor, you know that her fears are largely unfounded and you have to work diligently to convince her of that. Luckily for you, the same social proof and collective ignorance fueling her fears can be used to turn the tide in your favour.

Social proof, or social influence, is when people choose to perform an action that they believe is appropriate by gauging the actions of others in the same social situation, whom they assume know better. A psychological phenomenon, it is common in situations where a person is unfamiliar with the correct mode of behaviour and so relies on others for that information. It's particularly powerful when the others are believed to be especially knowledgeable, as is the case with "experts."

We refer to this phenomenon as "following the herd," a type of conformity that results in people selecting a single choice, even if a person does not believe it is correct.

You have multiple opportunities to use social influence to your advantage. Once the patient satisfies her own curiosity through forums, blogs, and other mediums, she'll turn to your site for more information. This is where you can use your patients to help further the social influence effect. Getting written testimonials and putting them onto the site is a great way of showcasing what your patients say. The same goes with testimonials and video stories. Why not write up the whole experience from your patient's perspective into a patient story?

There are some jurisdictions in which testimonials are strictly prohibited because of government guidelines regarding advertising of private medical practices. However, that doesn't mean you can't have social proof. Use your imagination and think of ways to put prospects in front of patients. One example is adding your Facebook feed on your site so people can see how many others like your page and are engaging with your practice. You're only limited by your imagination.

6. **Determination:** *When she makes a firm decision to do something about her condition*

Action is born of thought but not all thoughts are the same.

"In any situation, the best thing you can do is the right thing;
the next best thing you can do is the wrong thing;
the worst thing you can do is nothing."
—Theodore Roosevelt

Determination is a higher state of mind. It's a driver for change and it's a gateway to action. The person that's **determined** to do something, will do it no matter the consequences. The person that *decides* to do something is just as likely to sit and watch TV all night.

It's the determined individual that you want to engage. It's up to you to provide a call to action that resonates with her determination and makes it easy for her to take the crucial actions that lead to booking a procedure with you.

7. Action: *The concrete first step on the road to the close*

Action only occurs when your prospective patient takes action on her mental decision. Up to this point, the process has only existed in her mind. You've had no way of knowing who she was or that she's been secretly courting your practice. This is the step where most physicians get it all wrong, to the point where I've seen hundreds of thousands of marketing dollars and effort go to waste. How you handle the first point of contact can make or break your business.

Step seven is the pivotal juncture on the Buying Roadmap. Think of it as a fork in the road. Your patient needs to decide to go to you or take the other path to your competitor, or worse yet, to do nothing. She's spent hours researching you and reading your site. You've built rapport with her digitally in text and video. But there is no way to know if you have traction unless the rubber meets the road.

Your client is ready to raise her hand, and there are three primary ways she may choose to enter your business.

a) Telephone

The phone is still by far the most common way patients will want to reach you. Many pundits and consultants will say that the phone is dying and email is king but I've found that to be far from the truth. Any examination of a tactical device, such as a telephone, needs to revert right back to the cognitive psychology of the user.

Your patient is in a vulnerable state. She's trying to solve a deeply personal issue. She cares about her appearance and has a high degree of caring about the opinion of others. She's not looking for convenience; she's looking for connection. The telephone is the most effective way of comfortably connecting and it also affords immediate gratification. There is no waiting for a reply or wondering if her deeply personal issue got caught in a spam filter. The phone lead is also typically more serious and ready to commit. You'll get some tire kickers on the phone, but the likelihood is that there will be fewer than with email due to the more personal connection and higher effort exerted for the exchange.

Because the phone is your primary source of communication, it means that it, and the person answering it, are the two most expensive things in your office. Why?

As a savvy practice owner, you may have spent tens of thousands of dollars on your site, on Google ads, and print advertising. You pour a lot into your promotions, and rightly so. All those marketing dollars have no other purpose than to drive a call to your practice. That call could have cost you as much as $1,000, depending on the medium. If you start looking at every lead call along those lines, you can see why that phone is so valuable. Now let's look at why it can be expensive.

In the average practice, I see little to no attention being paid to how the phone is handled. Most doctors don't track their incoming calls. They don't record the calls for quality and they don't mystery shop their practice. This means that they're flying blind. Do you know how many of your calls go to voicemail and then get hung up before the person leaves a message? Do you know if your receptionist is saying the right things on the call? Is she picking up every call that comes in? If your answer is *no* and you feel bad, that's good. Use that pain to make a change and improve the situation.

Now let's assume that the calls are being picked up. The second biggest issue I see is that the frontline receptionist has little-to-no training in sales or handling objections. Most doctors put someone in front of the phone, give her general directions, and hope for the best.

Do you REALLY know how your receptionists are handling your incoming calls?

Do you remember Wile E. Coyote and The Roadrunner? No matter how hard that coyote ran, he could never get through the black hole painted on the side of that stone wall. Some receptionists are exactly like that. They're the immovable, or incompetent, force that turns your hard work and money into a big, painful joke.

Your receptionist is the single most valuable person in your practice where new leads are concerned. As the ambassador for your office, your receptionist makes the first connection and her level of professionalism, empathy, and caring are part of the proof your prospect is looking for. At this point, it doesn't matter what you said online or what a prospect has seen of you on television. This is where the rubber meets the road. This is where she finds out if you're everything that she hoped for, or not, in which case she'll just be revving in neutral. Nothing makes a prospect lose trust more quickly than getting her call picked up by an ill-prepared, cranky, unsympathetic receptionist.

If you have a high no-show rate for consultations or a poor booking conversion rate on your incoming calls, you should start your investigations at the front desk and the telephone.

By the way, do you know your call-to-conversion rate? Do you track how many calls you get, how many get picked up, and how many convert to a consultation booking? If not, you should.

"Measurement is the first step that leads to control and eventually to improvement. If you can't measure something, you can't understand it. If you can't understand it, you can't control it. If you can't control it, you can't improve it."
—H. James Harrington

b) Email

Although I spent some of the previous section knocking down email, please don't get the impression that I think email is bad. It's a fabulous medium, but it's just not your primary medium.

Email has several advantages versus the telephone. It feels private. It allows for silent communication during work hours and it has the convenience of being used at your own pace.

Unfortunately, it's very easy to get email wrong. Here are some general tips and strategies you can use to ensure you have world-class email communication.

- Have an email form on your site and whitelist the incoming address so all your emails get through. Have a policy of checking all your spam filters four times a day. After all, if email isn't getting to you, you can't respond.

- Have enough staff to handle incoming email promptly. If you can get your response time down to under five minutes, it's great. A quick response time shows patients that you're receptive, professional, and that you care about them. This impression carries through to the entire treatment process. In addition to staff, it helps to have your marketing manager write out appropriate email boilerplates that can be easily reused by the staff. This way you ensure accurate and professional communication no matter who's working that day.

- Don't treat email like a second-rate medium. Give it the same respect as you would your phone, because even though email leads may be slightly less frequent, they cost just as much to generate.

When your patient first emails you, its content does not cover the full context. She may be asking about price and availability but her subconscious is ever vigilant and looking out for the proof of your claims. Responding quickly tells her subconscious that if she has a problem, she can easily get in touch with your office. A two- to three-day response time tells her that it may be just as hard to get in touch with you during an emergency. *How* you say something can mean even more than *what* you say. We're all logical and emotional creatures. There is no way to separate how we feel from what we think. It's imperative that you pay attention to both.

c) Social Media

In a cosmetic surgery practice, the social media contact is going to be your least frequent contact method. However, this medium has some unique properties of which you need to be aware.

The phone calls and emails you receive are meant to be private and discreet communications between your office and your patient. Social media is a different animal, primarily in that it's a public conversation. Everything you do on your Facebook page is visible to the entire online community. How you handle everything, from a lead to a complaint, is judged and scrutinised by everyone in that community. This means that being prompt and addressing every interaction becomes pivotal to your success. Something you did two months ago lingers on your social media page and is easily found by just scrolling down.

The upside to the public scrutiny is that you now get a double bonus of leverage and social proof. How you handle the communication stays on your page so other prospects can make a decision about you. They may not contact you publicly, but they can use their newly found impression to take the step of calling or emailing you. The other major benefit you get is the social proof. If someone asks about booking a consultation online, they're showing others that they're willing to do business with you. The herd mentality kicks in and you get the benefit of unsolicited endorsement. This is the time to run promotions, regular but infrequent. Make them special and truly worth talking about. Because people like you and pay attention to you, you're much more likely to start converting your list to sales.

With social media, you should ideally try to get your response time down to about two minutes. It's an instant medium and needs ongoing attention.

8. Defence of Choice

In the sales world, it's often said that people buy on emotion, not logic. It's the basis for countless sales courses and books, but they all have it wrong. If you ignore logic and reason, you're cutting yourself short and leaving a ton of money on the table.

The reality is that your sales job doesn't end in the office. While I agree that emotion is a huge motivator in the decision-making process, I'm also keenly aware of the fact that people don't buy in a bubble.

When a woman makes the decision to go through with surgery, whether for emotional or logical reasons, she then has to defend her decision to the other people in her life. Everyone from family and friends to spouses and partners need a reason to agree with her choice. She may have made the decision to go with you, but there may be an army of detractors waiting to talk her out of it as soon as she gets home.

Defending her choice is not always easy and it's up to

you to provide the tools, weapons, and ammunition she needs to win those arguments. You have to make the logical case for her decision to go through with her surgery. You'll need to provide written answers and scientific proof that her procedure is safe and that you're the right surgeon for the job, prepared in a complete consultation package that she can bring home and review in private. She can then use that information to disarm all those in her life who disapprove, and more importantly, may prevent you from getting the sale.

I call this phase the "After Sale," and something you should put in place and work to constantly refine.

You might be tempted to tell me that you already have a package that goes home with your patients. Before you do, go back and ask yourself these questions:

Does my package give my patient all the help she needs to defend her decision to go through with a cosmetic procedure or surgery?

Does my package credential me and reassure a third party that might be reviewing me and my profile for competence and expertise?

Does my package position me as a specialist in the field and leader in the procedures being evaluated?

Does my package give a clear next step for the patient to get started?

Does my package provide answers to every and all

possible objections a spouse or family member might use to talk my patient out of the surgery?

If the answer is anything other than a resounding *YES* to the above, you need to go back and do some work on your After-Sale process.

9. Commitment

Something interesting happens in our brains when we pay for something. Until that point, the possibility of purchasing and going through with a procedure is about fifty-fifty. Anything can tip the scales and cause abandonment, no matter how well you've done everything along the way. Before they put their money down, you're just another doctor and all options are still open.

But the moment your patient pays for surgery, her mind changes to complete commitment. Cognitive dissonance kicks in and she begins to firmly and strongly defend her choice. No other doctor will do and she won't want to listen to anyone telling her she's made the wrong choice.

For most patients, that's what goes on and your surgery simply moves ahead without incident. However, there is a second situation which needs careful fostering. For some patients, worry kicks in and they can experience extreme anxiety before surgery. Most patients get nervous, but it's the extreme cases that need to be managed.

For the record, you should never use tactics and tricks

to get a woman to go through with surgery against her wishes. I'm working under the assumption that you've taken every ethical precaution to make sure that this is the right decision for her and that it's safe to proceed with surgery. In fact, the surgery is going to alleviate a lot of issues for her and it's in her best interest to continue. For this kind of patient, you have to eliminate the self-sabotage that can lead to an abandoned surgery.

The typical surgeon, and his staff, simply stops selling as soon as the paperwork is signed. He doesn't call the patient again and nobody follows up with her until shortly before her surgery, but that's a mistake.

You should have a predefined set of emails that go out to a patient in a steady flow leading up to her surgery. We refer to this as a drip sequence.

You should send out information on what she should be doing, what to eat and not to eat, why she made the right decision, and how excited she's going to be with her new body once it's all over. You have to reassure your patient every step of the way. Make her feel cared for and appreciated. Let her feel that she made the right decision. Setting up some videos where you explain things can further enhance the experience and strengthen the bond.

Don't make the assumption that the surgery is guaranteed. Work to keep your patients happy and calm. It will pay dividends after the surgery and when it comes time to sell her additional services after her recovery. It will a generate referrals and glowing online reviews.

10. Justification

The time after surgery is when most problems can arise regarding patient satisfaction and getting referrals. Right after surgery, there is a lot of pain, regret, and the inevitable "I told you so" from people in the patient's life who were against the surgery to begin with (and were just waiting to prove you, and her, wrong). This volatile time can and should be managed as carefully as you manage the healing and recovery of her surgery.

The process of containing potentially negative issues after surgery and enhancing the patient experience starts before surgery. In the days and weeks leading up to her surgery, she should receive clear descriptions of what she's likely to experience coupled with social proof from others that have gone through it. If you can get other patients to appear on short video clips talking about their surgery day, pain, and recovery, all the better. These private videos can be made available online through a patient portal on your website and dripped out to the new patient in a carefully orchestrated email sequence.

You can further enhance the outcome by managing expectations. The worst thing you can do is overpromise and underdeliver. It's much better to set lower expectations and overdeliver. If she gets a little more than she was expecting or a little less pain, she'll think you're a phenomenal surgeon. If, however, you promise no pain and she is in even a little bit of pain, you'll look like an amateur. Manage her expectations and you'll be managing your degree of future success.

Post-surgery is also the time when you have to look out for buyer's remorse.

Buyer's remorse is the sense of regret after having made a purchase. It's frequently associated with the purchase of an expensive item such as a car or house. It may stem from fear of making the wrong choice, guilt over extravagance, or a suspicion of having been overly influenced by the seller.[2]

I'm assuming that you don't employ sleazy sales tactics and false scarcity or undue pressure to close a sale so we won't go into that. In cosmetic patients, buyer's remorse is caused by pain and guilt. You can manage the pain with medications and setting expectations as described above, but the guilt is another matter.

Some women feel guilty that they spent a lot of money on themselves when they have kids and obligations. They might even be made to feel guilty by parents or judgmental friends and co-workers. It's important that your entire team reassures her of having made the right decision for herself and all the reasons that she deserves to have something positive in her life and just for her. Most women are conditioned by society to be selfless when it comes to their family. You need to overcome that preconditioning and let her enjoy doing something to improve her overall appearance, confidence, and state of mind. The truth is that many women feel empowered by their new body, and all the people in their lives benefit from this new and rejuvenated mental state. It's often in her very best interest to have surgery with a competent physician who will give her meaningful and lasting results.

The Buying Roadmap is one of the primary pillars to the Practice Growth Formula. Unfortunately, the scope of this book is not to discuss every single tactic we employ. However, it's my hope that you'll take the 10 steps of the Buying Roadmap and use them as a measuring stick of your own efforts. Use them to brainstorm ideas. Start implementing new marketing initiatives for each of the steps to walk a patient into your waiting room and successfully grow your practice.

If They Don't Believe You, They Don't Buy. And They Don't Believe You.

THE IMPORTANCE OF CREDENTIALING OR ABC

There's a saying they used to teach salespeople back in the day of the hard close. They called it the ABC of sales: Always Be Closing. Those greasy old-style hard-close tactics are no longer used, but the adage still applies. In today's atmosphere, we take a less direct approach and help the patient come to her own conclusion. We educate her and allow her to make a decision at her pace. But make no mistake about it, your job is still to close. Every word on your website, every post on your Facebook page, and everything you say on the phone is designed for one purpose: to help her choose to have surgery with you.

If you truly believe that you're the best surgeon and that going to someone else wouldn't be in your prospect's best interest, you have a moral and an ethical obligation to help her choose you over any and all competitors in the market. Your only job, then, is to make sure you deliver on your promises.

CREDENTIALING IS KEY

Credentialing is integral to the closing process. It sets you up as the authority figure in the consultation. It reassures the patient about her choices and allows you to take control of the consultation and closing process.

In 1961, the Yale University psychologist, Dr. Stanley Milgram, conducted a series of experiments on authority and obedience. Participants were asked to take the role of a "teacher" and were placed in a room with a shock generator marked with levels from 15 to 450 volts, to which a "student" was hooked up in another room. The participant, as the "teacher," presented a series of questions to the "student," and with each incorrect response, they were ordered to deliver a shock of increasing intensity to the point that they were painful but not dangerous. As the experiment progressed, the "student" would complain about a heart condition, plead to be released, and reacted increasingly more violently, until he finally refused to respond and fell completely silent. The majority of participants asked the experimenter if they should continue, to which the response was always the same:

1. "Please continue."
2. "The experiment requires that you continue."
3. "It is absolutely essential that you continue."
4. "You have no other choice; you must go on."

Sixty-five percent of participants delivered the maximum voltage of 450, despite hearing the tortured reaction of their "students." (Interestingly, 84 percent were glad to have taken part in the study, and only 1 percent regretted it.)

More recent research has shown that the presence of authority can actually shut down some of the brain's cognitive functions. One Danish study involved scanning the brains of Pentecostalists listening to recorded prayers delivered by three groups: non-Christians, "ordinary" Christians, and a healer. When the participants were told that they would be listening to the healer, the region of the brain involved in skepticism and vigilance shut down (portions of the prefrontal and anterior cingulate cortices). The researchers of the study suggest that similar deactivation may occur when listening to physicians, parents, and other charismatic leaders (Schjødt et al., 2009).

Your Sales Job Is Not Done Yet

By now you should have set up a unique and favourable position in the market. You should have highlighted your best credentials and educated your prospective patient on why you're the best choice. The time has come to take that all important booking call and have her come in for her consultation. You've done all the right things, and now she's in your waiting room. Should your staff still credential you? Absolutely!

It's the combination of credibility and likeability that needs to occur in order to build trust. And trust is essential for the close. In today's world of ever-increasing media where people are bombarded with messages all day long, it's more important than ever to reinforce your own position and recreate that trust. Credentialing should be done by your staff on the call and the initial consultation. Positioning you as the authority in your field just before the patient's consultation will reinforce your ability to benevolently influence her towards a positive decision. Your website, your phone scripts, your staff, and ultimately *you* should ALWAYS BE CLOSING. It's the ultimate goal of your marketing machine. There is no other purpose to its existence.

"The purpose of business is to create and keep a customer."
—Peter F. Drucker

DON'T WALLOW IN MEDIOCRITY

Spend a lot of time on a few great things. Doing more is not the way to get more. Being mediocre at ten things is not nearly as good as being gifted at one. People don't buy from generalists.

There are three main levels to earning income as a physician:

1. Generalist
2. Specialist
3. Celebrity

In any profession you examine, those will be the main levels of earning income. The medical profession is no exception.

A plastic surgeon or neurosurgeon makes more than a general practitioner (GP). The Specialist has much more earning capacity than a Generalist. A Specialist is looked at as someone with additional training, experience, and specialised skill in an area. For that reason, he can command more money. **It doesn't matter how good you are; all that matters is how you're perceived.** When you position your online persona, it should give the reader every indication that you're the authority in the field, that you're the go-to person for the service you provide. This can sometimes mean that you'll refuse to do other kinds of surgeries and focus on sucking in all the business for your primary one or two procedures. For example, if you're good at breasts and tummies, you want to pull in all the available business in that category. This means that all your online positioning should make the patient feel that you're the only person that can possibly give her the results she wants—that you do this day in and day out and that you know your stuff better than your competitors.

Think about it like this: If you owned a classic Porsche and it needed repairs, would you go to a local mechanic down the street, a mechanic that specializes in classic cars, or a mechanic that specializes only in classic Porsches? Chances are that you wouldn't trust your pride and joy to anyone but a Specialist, and it's no different for a patient looking to enhance her body.

Being a Specialist positions you for an exponential increase in income. You'll be able to capture more of the market, charge more for your services, and eliminate most buying resistance associated with a Generalist positioning.

The Celebrity is the next level up. It takes more work and you have to publish a book as well as make countless public appearances, but being a Celebrity will increase your earning potential even further. Examples of Celebrities are Dr. Phil and Dr. Oz. Both of them can achieve a higher earning potential than they could as a Generalist.

However, you don't need to become a media whore to reap some of the benefits of Celebrity status, even in your position as a Specialist, because it can be easily bought. You can associate yourself with the Celebrity level even if you've never been one yourself and have no desire to be. There are any number of professional actors who were once famous and aren't in the business anymore. These actors can be signed up for a relatively low sum of money or perhaps even in exchange for services to represent your practice. You can negotiate their endorsement and then use their fame to propel yourself slightly beyond the Specialist arena.

When choosing your celebrity model, you should consider her credibility and how she resonates with your target audience. Just because someone is more famous doesn't mean she's more credible. Purchasing celebrity endorsement is surprisingly affordable, and it's an avenue you can consider pursuing once you have all your other positioning elements lined up.

At first, focus all your effort on elevating yourself above the other plastic surgeons and demonstrate that you're the foremost authority for the procedures and services you want to offer. Have the courage to cut out the deadwood and focus on the surgeries that bring you the most money and most satisfaction for the least number of hassles and complications. Once you become the Specialist, you won't need to scrounge for every single procedure you might know how to do. You'll do what you love and bank the profit from it.

Show, Don't Tell

One of the biggest misconceptions about marketing is the attitude that saying something is the same as proving something.

I see ineffectual marketing all over the medical industry, with doctors touting their concern for aesthetic quality and how they're artists at surgery. Do you think the patients believe it? Not for a second!

Saying something without proving it is little more than hype. *Hyperbole*, by definition, is described as exaggerated statements or claims not meant to be taken literally.

> *"What you do speaks so loudly that I cannot hear what you say."*
> —Ralph Waldo Emerson

We've all been trained from childhood to distrust salesmen. The average person is hardwired to assume they're being cheated. Think about how you feel every time a medical sales rep tries to corner you at a convention to sell you the latest piece of gear that's supposed to make you millions. You probably react immediately and instinctively by putting your guard up and saying no to pretty much every request he or she makes. You've been sold equipment that didn't work well. And, I bet not a single rep showed you how to fill your waiting room with people who want to take advantage of this latest gadget you just bought.

Your prospective patients are just as skeptical about you as you feel about medical sales reps. The way to get around this is the universal concept of proof. Show, don't tell.

If you feel you're at an artistic level of mastery in your field, you need to prove it to the patient. Everything, from how your before-and-after photos are displayed to your waiting room and personal attire, speaks volumes. Patients make a judgment call about what you're saying based on the very first interaction they have with you. If you don't have before-and-after pictures on your site, they may think you have something to hide. If you won't let them speak to other clients or offer testimonials, again, they have nothing compelling to persuade them that your perceived hype is truth.

When it comes time to show and not tell, you need to start thinking of the experience of engaging with you and your brand as a tipping scale. Every proof element you provide helps the scales reach the tipping point from doubt to certainty, from disbelief to desire. Every pebble of proof you provide to support your written and spoken statements contributes positively to increasing your conversion rate both online and during your consultation.

Here are some areas you should pay close attention to when you want to start doing more than talking about how good you are.

YOUR WEBSITE

Is it aesthetically pleasing? Does it have a professional appearance created for you by a design expert or is it something you put together yourself? What you might think is good is not necessarily what sells. Is your writing informative and correct in both grammar and tone? Did you have your content checked for spelling mistakes and accuracy? Did you test your website to prove that it resonates with your audience and converts visitors to patients? Did you test the conversion rate for the design? Are you tracking the number of patients who make it to your contact page, and are you working to improve that number on an ongoing basis?

YOUR BEFORE-AND-AFTER PHOTOS

Before-and-after images should be of the highest quality. They're essentially your artist's portfolio and one of the biggest reasons people will choose you over the competition. Assuming you do great work, you need to set up a system for gaining consistency. You should make sure that all your photos are in focus (you'd be surprised how often I've seen blurry photos used), have consistent lighting, and are on the same solid-coloured background. Make sure that any facial images are taken without makeup both in the before and after. Remember that your prospective client is naturally skeptical. She's looking for anything to warn her that the image is doctored or not the same person. Being consistent and makeup-free with perfect clarity gives you the best chance at being believed. You want patients focused on your work, not on the quality of the photo or any tricks that might have been employed.

YOUR WAITING ROOM

Your waiting room is the gateway to a positive sales process. It's the first impression the patient has of the physical interaction with your practice. Until now, all her experiences have been virtual. The waiting room and front desk are where you start to gain traction. It's there where the real work of making her fall in love with your practice really begins. Waiting rooms are a microcosm of activity, with everything from phones ringing at reception to patients paying for their treatment.

I look at the waiting room from the perspective of *elastic time*. I'm no physicist, but I do know how patients think. In the human mind, time is not constant. Or more accurately, the perception of time is not constant. It can be stretched or contracted based on the activity in which the patient engages.

Think back to a time you were having a really great conversation with a friend or new romantic interest. Remember how time used to fly by? Hours would flash past as if you were not on the same plane of existence you were on before meeting, when you were just waiting for and anticipating the encounter. How we perceive time is infinitely variable, and it's this perception of time that dictates the quality of the experience in your waiting room.

It's not always easy to fix the logistical processes that lead to longer or shorter wait times. Sometimes, a patient may talk too long and you just can't get out for the next appointment in time. It happens to everyone. It doesn't mean you shouldn't try to be punctual but it does mean that you should have a process that *plan* kicks in when things are running behind.

The best way to reduce the perception of time is to engage your prospects, mind and body, in an activity. Something as simple as proactively serving a drink (and snacks) and engaging the person in light conversation can make all the difference.

It's the same reason that mirrors are commonly found in

elevators. With the construction of high-rises following World War II, passengers frequently complained about elevator delays. However, with the installation of mirrors, complaints decreased dramatically because it gave passengers something to do, which made their wait feel shorter.

Think of all the ways you can positively engage the patient in the waiting room, because the worst thing you can do is let them sit there idly listening to canned music, or worse, the local radio station. (I was standing in a client's full waiting room once and the receptionist had the local radio station on, when a commercial for a competing surgeon started playing. It was great advertising, but not for my client!)

Most times waiting rooms are just boring places to sit, and that's the standard expectation.

What are you doing to make your waiting room a pleasant and engaging experience to defy the standard?

YOUR PERSONAL OFFICE

Your office is your domain. It should be designed as a tool for conversion. You should stop thinking of it as a place where you do paperwork and meet patients and start thinking of it as the single biggest opportunity you have to convert a prospect into a patient. Your office has only one purpose when it comes to business growth: to carefully build trust and credibility so the patient believes what you're saying and begins to like you.

Your office is where the job of influence and relationship-building blossom. You should make sure the environment is professional but not cold. This is the place to display all your credentials and accolades. Make sure to add personal touches that make you seem more human and approachable. You have to strike a fine balance between being likable and being respected.

I've seen doctors' offices that ranged from messy to extremely cold. The only decoration on one office wall I visited was a golf certificate—that's not what you want the patient to think you're doing with your time and her money! Every single item in your office contributes or detracts from your ability to close that surgical sale. Take thirty minutes with a notebook and sit in the chair your patients sit in. What do they see? What are they thinking? How can you improve it? Make notes and make changes and you'll reap the benefit with higher closing rates and more money in your bank account.

CHAPTER 5

Positioning for Success

The Battle Is Fought in the Mind, Not Online

A war is being fought in your prospect's mind. A constant pull and push between emotion, logic, reason, and desire. She brings new ammunition to the battle every time she visits a web page. She arms herself with new information from your site or one of your competitor's. She searches for truth and understanding. She wants proof of your abilities and she's looking for a reason to let you win that war. She'll find some ease once she fills out your online consultation booking form, but she won't find peace until she makes a final decision and puts down her deposit for surgery.

WIN BY GIVING WHAT YOUR PATIENT WANTS

Let's look at Sony's Betamax videocassette, more commonly referred to as Beta. Beta was better than VHS in many ways. It was smaller so it cost less to ship; it had better picture quality so the consumer got a higher quality experience; and filmmakers got to show off their creations properly. It was more stable and lasted longer. It had every reason to win at the war of business, but did it succeed? No. It failed because quality has absolutely nothing to do with success.

JVC out-maneuvered Sony and gave the consumer what he was asking for, longer home-recording times being one of them. The "perceived value" of the longer recording time eventually tipped the scale, and Beta died a quiet death all over the world.

The battle for supremacy took place in the consumer's mind. VHS managed to establish a strong foothold in their consumers' minds, which allowed people to dig in and plant their flag firmly in that camp. Choosing VHS had nothing to do with quality. It became a sensible and rational financial decision. It let people feel like they were making the *prudent* choice, the sensible and practical choice that any intelligent person would make. Kids all over the world got pats on the head for calculating the play time of VHS versus Beta and parroting back the same limiting beliefs that they were taught by their parents: the belief that cheaper saves money. It didn't matter that they were paying less and getting less—less quality, less enjoyment. They got the *feeling* of more. And that's all it took for VHS to dominate and win the race.

It's not about the real world. It's about your prospect's mindset. Perception is reality and it has huge financial implications for your practice.

If you have nothing setting you apart from your competition; if you give her no reason to come to <u>*you*</u>; if you don't give her something she can stand on and the ability to defend her decision to friends, family and co-workers, and even to herself, you're just one of many insignificant and irrelevant choices. It's not her fault she didn't choose you. It's yours. Take responsibility for that and take action towards crafting a unique and defendable position in your market.

You can't usually rush creating a position. This kind of positioning takes me anywhere from six to sixty hours of interviewing a client to get to the core essence of what makes him unique. I've been doing this for a long time and I know what I'm looking for, and it still takes time to do it right. It may take you longer. Don't despair, and keep at it until you have something that will suck business out of your competitor's hands and place it firmly into yours.

IT'S NOT WHAT YOU SAY, IT'S WHAT THEY WANT TO HEAR

The way in which something is presented makes all the difference to how it will be received. Your patients want to hear things in a way that makes them comfortable and matches their state of mind. It's not about what *you* want to say. It's all about what they're minds are open to hearing.

For example, a youth shelter wouldn't be nearly as supported by a community or donors if it were called *Hoodlum Housing*. *The Charity for the Poor* wouldn't be funded if it were referred to as

The Organisation for the Continuation of the Victim Mentality. Everything, from how you name your business to how you position your procedures, creates a predisposition in the cognitive centres of your patient's mind. *The Institute for Advanced Cosmetic Surgery* is different from *The Institute for Safe Cosmetic Surgery.* Just one word can completely alter the perception of a practice. The former will attract a buyer looking for new techniques while the latter may appeal to someone for whom safety is the overriding concern. Words matter. What you say matters. How you string your words together matters. It all works together to create a position in the patient's mind—a position that can help or hinder your efforts at financial, personal, and emotional success.

HOW POSITIONING WORKS IN THE MIND

Dr. Smith Plastic Surgeon will be perceived very differently from *The Smith Centre for Physical Beauty.* Each position sets up camp in your prospect's mind. She then automatically and immediately associates characteristics to your practice based on past experience. Every encounter she's had with a medical office and big brand sets up cognitive predispositions, which your brand can then take advantage of, or has to fight against.

We're all products of the conditioning we received as children. What was done by our parents, grandparents, and teachers is then enhanced and augmented by society. Popular culture, collective intelligence/stupidity, and media all play a role in our belief system. Your patients are a walking collection of all they were conditioned to think—a veritable alchemic mixture of beliefs, which you can use to create gold if you know the right formula.

The same predispositions that influence thought are true at the procedure level. A *chemical peel* sounds very different from a *topical skin restoration treatment.* The first sounds like an industrial accident. The second sounds like a good idea.

Don't assume that you should be using the industry standard terminology. There is a time and a place to follow, and another when you should lead. You must take advantage of the way your prospective patient thinks and leverage industry education efforts for your own ends.

Don't, however, make the mistake of thinking that I'm advocating one approach over another with regards to naming procedures (like in the previous paragraphs). My goal is simply to make you aware of how and what you're saying, and how that's being perceived and framed in your patients' minds. Every approach you take needs to be safely and carefully tested. You have to evaluate your competition and then set up the language patterns and position that give you a unique advantage in the marketplace. Most important of all, the new position you create has to be believable and accepted by your prospective patient. You should never change the name of a service for the simple sake of standing out. It should be attached to a greater strategic objective.

Think of people's decision process as them putting choices in mental baskets. They generalize, and compartmentalize, so they can more easily cope with the barrage of information they're given. Your only job is to make it easy for her to place all your competitors in the same basket: the waste basket.

This has to be done for you, your practice, your services, and even your staff. All facets of your practice need to be positioned in such a way that the consumer has one clear choice to make, and that choice is you. Leave no room for ambiguity or unsupervised thought on the part of the prospect. Control every aspect of how you're seen and what opinions people form about you. Give them the logical arguments they need in order to defend their choices and the emotional connection required to bond to you and your practice on a deeper level.

Multiple Levels of Positioning

Positioning isn't something you do once and forget about. It's not something that should only be done for you or your practice on a broad level. There are many levels of positioning and you need to pay attention to them all. Your prospect is not making one decision. She's making a series of small decisions along her buying journey, all to which you need her to say yes. Let's examine the different levels of positioning in the sequence that your prospect is likely to engage, starting at the ad level and moving all the way up to the practice level.

POSITIONING YOUR PPC ADS

Positioning at the micro level can, and should, be applied to your online ads. While you only have a couple of sentences to make an impact, how you position the ad against the competing ads can dramatically influence the click-through rate, cost, and ROI.

For example, here are a few headline options for ad titles:

Larger Breasts
Get Larger Breasts
The Breast Expert
Increase Self-Confidence
Get the Look You Want
Get the Look You Deserve
Leading Breast Surgeon

Which of those ad titles do you think will perform best? Don't know? That's okay, neither do I. The truth is that there's no way to know until you start testing, and only after you've examined what the competition is doing. The worst thing is to make your ad an "also-ran." You need your ad to stand out. If you were going against those ads, here are a few you could try, assuming your positioning was honest and matched the messaging.

Zero-Risk Breast Surgery
99%-Safe Breast Surgery
Surgeon to the Stars
Guaranteed Surgery

All those titles have a unique advantage and position against the previous ads. Whether they work or not needs to be tested and is largely irrelevant at this point. What I'm after is getting you to think about your ads in this way—to look at the competition and your prospect and give her an ad that matches her psychology, while simultaneously positioning you to win the click. Google will always serve three ads at the top of search results. You don't always have to be #1 to win the click, but you do have to be the ad that best positions against the others shown. By being more interesting, provocative, or advantageous, you can win clicks even when in the second and third position.

Look at your PPC campaigns and start testing and tracking changes. PPC is the fastest way to get into the mind of your prospect and get concrete evidence of their psyche, which you can then apply to all your marketing, online and offline.

POSITIONING YOUR PRACTICE

Your practice position is the macro-level positioning. It encompasses your "brand" as a whole and defines what your practice stands for. It's the bird's eye view of your company and what people can expect. But it's not the most important because your patient is not buying your brand; she's buying a result.

Being a standout practice takes a lot of effort. You have to do things in a way that others are not willing to do. You have to create an _experience_. You have to slowly build a brand, which takes time, money, and effort. Luckily for you, it's not the most important aspect you need to pay attention to. In fact, if you get the rest right, positioning your practice will come naturally as an evolution of positioning the rest of your micro-level differentiators.

POSITIONING YOUR PROCEDURES

Many surgeons assume that the patient is interested in their practice, and that's why they spend a lot of time focusing on branding the practice, while completely ignoring the procedures.

Unless you're a huge corporation with far-reaching needs, building a brand is a waste of your time. Without a multimillion-dollar budget, brands are born, they're not built. If you do everything else right, your practice will evolve into a brand. And by brand, I don't mean a consistent logo and look—that's called an identity system and you should always invest in that. I'm talking about the emotive and visceral attributes associated with your company. However, that's not something you need to worry about now. The single most important positioning element you need to undertake is for your procedure.

Your prospective patient is looking for a reason to break you out of the commodity death trap. She's looking for some kind of benefit or fear alleviation to use as a reason to come to your practice instead of your competitor's. She's yearning for something to stake her hopes on and justify it to the other people in her life. That job falls entirely on you.

Positioning your procedures is all about examining what you're doing and seeing how it differs from your competition. If you use a special tool that gives you better results, you need to make a big deal out of it and teach the client why it's better for her. For example, if you use custom anesthesia protocols, you have to tell her about them.

Every surgeon that does quality work does something his

colleagues don't. You're probably no different. The only problem is that nobody knows about it.

People can't appreciate of what they're not aware. Your special skills, techniques, and instruments need to be brought out of the operating room and into the light of day. It's up to you to show people what you do. They're not going to guess at it, and they have no way of knowing to ask about it.

HOW TO POSITION YOURSELF AND YOUR PROCEDURES

Positioning your procedures correctly will give you the single biggest advantage in your marketing. It gives your patients a reason to choose you over the other doctors in town, and it will start giving you the money you need to begin the second phase of the Practice Growth Formula.

While positioning is as much art as science, here is a systematic way you can start the process of positioning your services.

Step 1—Interview and Research

Positioning starts with an earnest evaluation of your competitors. You can't know how to differentiate yourself until you know in what way you need to be different. Your first step is to go to all of your competitors' sites and note what they're saying about themselves and their procedures, what information they're providing and what their angle is. One of them might be offering a twenty-four-hour-recovery breast augmentation, or perhaps a drain-free tummy tuck. Whatever it is, you need to look at them and honestly identify what it is that makes you stand out.

Once you have your notes, ask a friend, spouse, or staff member to interview you about what you do and why you do it. Go deep into your procedure to the technical level. Make them hold you to task if there is something they didn't understand. Make sure you go through the entire operation, from the pre-surgical assessment to suturing and postoperative care.

There are hidden gems in everything you do, which are either special and unique, or which your colleagues failed to communicate. Even if you do everything in the exact same way as your competitor, the simple fact that you say it first and frame it in a positive light will give you an edge in the prospect's mind.

Step 2—Identification

Now that you have your notes from the research and your interview, it's time to identify the qualities you want to communicate. Go through your list of items and pull out all the things you do that are different or that your competitors are not communicating.

From that list, pull out any items that would give the patient an advantage—anything that will either enhance her result, reduce the risk of the surgery, or give her a more positive experience overall. This list is the master list of attributes you'll use to build your position.

Step 3—Position

Take your list and examine the current procedure pages on your website. Are you communicating all those positive attributes?

If not, start doing so. Rewrite pages and clearly communicate the features and benefits of what you do for the patient. Show her why your procedure is better and give her a reason to choose you.

When selecting the attributes, try to put yourself in the patient's frame of mind. She's interested in <u>results</u> and she has <u>fears</u>. Anything you can do to educate her on why things will be better and safer with you should go on your final write-up.

Step 4—Test

Most doctors would stop at step three and feel very proud of themselves. Truthfully, I'd be very happy if you implemented even to that level. But without testing, you're flying blindly into mediocrity. If you want to lead, you need to see where you are, and where you're going.

Once you have the final write-ups, you need to start testing your new pages against your existing content. Never abandon what you're doing before you know you have something better. You need to test for page engagement, site engagement, and how many people make it through to the next phase in the buying process, as well as how many people contact you or, at the very least, make it to your contact page.

Once you have the winning variation, you can either start again or start refining the winner to maximize the conversion.

Positioning yourself is no different. You have unique education, residency, and experience. Your personal life is filled with volunteer work and a childhood that nobody can replicate. You only need to dig into those aspects of your life and identify the advantageous and attractive attributes to highlight using the same four-step process outlined above.

Get the positioning right and you'll maximize the return on the existing marketing for which you're already paying. You'll get more from your PPC ads, more from your print ads, and more money to grow, all for spending not a dime more. Conversion is, quite literally, free money after the initial investment of your time.

CHAPTER 6

The Attraction Side of the Formula

Once you've done everything possible to increase your conversion, it's time to think about attraction. Combining conversion with attraction gives you the multiplier effect needed for meaningful and sustained growth.

When I speak of attraction, I'm talking about eyeballs on pages. There are many ways to acquire web traffic. While we do work with PPC, I find that an ongoing stream of unpaid web traffic yields an abundance of success for our clients.

Why Natural Search Engine Results Are More Powerful Than PPC

There are two ways to appear in a search engine result: PPC and natural/unpaid. Both have distinct advantages and disadvantages. From a positioning standpoint, natural/unpaid, or "organic," results have a certain psychological edge over pay-per-click campaigns.

When you pay for a PPC ad, a majority of users know that you're paying Google to be at the top. They look at it as a simple advertisement and nothing more. We're hardwired to think that advertising is misleading and dishonest, so while you may get a click, you're not getting the full positioning benefit of the organic listing.

Patients believe that the organic results are something produced by billions of dollars in research and countless PhDs at Google. They look at them as a sort of authoritative, unbiased result and you get to instantly leverage Google's credibility. Patients also look at those results as being the "best" in the category. They know that Google listens and watches and if the results are at the top, it's because most people find them useful. Google spends a lot of PR money making sure that people believe two things about them:

1. **They do no evil.**

2. **Their mission is to serve up the most useful and relevant content to their users.**

That incredible combination of authority, trust, and social proof is what makes an organic result so valuable. The simple "spend per click" from an organic result can't be calculated in comparison to PPC. You have to weigh in the psychological advantage of the positioning edge it gives you. Ranking highly on Google sets the user up to believe that you're credible and trustworthy. It makes your in-office conversion much smoother and helps turn sales calls into booking calls.

You've probably been told countless times that you should be online and pay attention to your rankings. I'm willing to bet, however, that nobody has ever explained the full implication of the psychology behind ranking and how it ripples across all your efforts. The reality is simple: you're not a complete authority until Google says you are.

In a 2010 interview with the *Telegraph* newspaper, Google's head of core ranking, Amit Singhal, said that Google is "the biggest kingmaker on this Earth."

Wikipedia says this:

> *Kingmaker is a term originally applied to the activities of Richard Neville, 16th Earl of Warwick — "Warwick the Kingmaker" — during the Wars of the Roses in England. The term has come to be applied more generally to a person or group that has great influence in a royal or political succession, without being a viable candidate.*[3]

A key part of your positioning strategy has to include solid online rankings. The good news is that if you know how to give Google what it wants, you will be King.

As important as your online ranking strategy is, it's still not where you should start. Remember, conversion trumps attraction. Get your positioning right and then go after Google. If you convert, you can afford to buy the Kingmaker's affections.

The King Needs Content

The phrase "content is king" is widely used in Internet marketing circles. It's a phrase that's completely true and wholly misunderstood. Content is only king if the reader *wants* to read it.

Your content strategy, and it has to be a strategy, should be designed around the Buying Roadmap, what the patient is thinking and the questions, concerns, and desires she may be expressing. Too often I see doctors throwing up content for the sake of adding pages to a site on the advice of a search-engine marketing "expert."

I'll state it plainly. Content for search engines is no different than content for marketing. You're not after stuffing key terms onto a page or trying to game the system. You're after the cognitive processes in your prospective patient's mind. If you systematically and strategically build out your content in volume, it will naturally be picked up and valued by search engines.

The single biggest problem with content development on cosmetic sites is the lack of a sustained effort. Most doctors look at their site as an event rather than a progression. They hire a company to put up a site once and then don't bother adding content in any meaningful way for years. Your site should be in a constant state of evolution. Once you get online, you need to feed the system as much quality content as you can, on an ongoing basis. This goes for your social media channels, your blog, and your main commercial website.

Remember, your site makes you money. If you have it converting well, it's in your best interest to drive as much targeted traffic to the site as possible.

Attraction Needs Multiple Sources

In the Practice Growth Formula, I state *T(ms)*: Traffic from multiple sources.

While focusing on search engines should always be your biggest concern, you need to understand that if you don't diversify, you're supporting your business infrastructure on a single pillar. Single-pillar roofs are never robust structures. If the search engines change things, or if you can't pay, your lead source dries up and so does your practice.

I had a client whose business was located on an island that was hit by major hurricanes a few years back. He was getting most of his business from Google-paid ads and a few other banner ad sources. When the hurricanes struck, his business was severely damaged. All his money had to go into repairs and many of them were not covered by insurance. His advertising money, literally, vanished overnight.

Luckily for him, he had just paid us to complete optimization work on his site. We got him ranking for his top key terms and the results of our work persisted, getting him business while he got his repairs completed. It carried him along until he was able to get the business profitable again, back on track, and paying for those PPC ads. We then encouraged him to get a Facebook page set up as an additional pillar of support. I'm happy to say that he's now thriving.

The point of that story is that you need to start thinking about the stability of your marketing before tragedy strikes. The more sources of traffic you have, the more stable your practice. The more stable your practice, the more certainty you'll have in future investments and expansion. Paying attention to the breadth and depth of your traffic sources is more important than any one key term.

CHAPTER 7

Strategy vs. Tactics

Strategy vs. Tactics

Never make a tactical move unless it furthers a strategic goal.

Wikipedia defines **strategy** as this:

... a high level plan to achieve one or more goals under conditions of uncertainty.

Strategy is important because the resources available to achieve these goals are usually limited.

Strategy is also about attaining and maintaining a position of advantage over adversaries through the successive exploitation of known or emergent possibilities rather than committing to any specific fixed plan designed at the outset.[4]

and **tactic** as this:

... a conceptual action implemented as one or more specific tasks."[5]

You should never make a tactical move if it doesn't further a strategic objective.

You're bombarded on a regular basis with information and advice regarding marketing, sales, business growth, medicine, and the like. It's easy to fall into the "what's new is what's important" trap. But don't implement that new 3D website widget because all your competitors are offering 3D education online.

I'm giving you permission to buck the trend and stop running around aimlessly. Imagine a general acting on every piece of intelligence and making his troops run around without a specific objective or aim. The results would be catastrophic.

To win, you have to take time and look ahead to your objective. You need to start with the end in mind and work backwards. A strategy is a high level plan for your success. It starts with your positioning and your objective. From there, you can then evaluate all your tactical options and decide if they further your goal or not. It also allows you to make the most effective use of your marketing dollars.

I don't want to just talk abstracts, so let's examine a real-world example of how strategy and tactics work.

Dr. Jones (not a real person, at least not one that I know) has some surgical capacity he'd like to fill with a new procedure. He's done some market research and shopped his competitors, discovering that butt augmentation is a lucrative opportunity and a rising trend due to recent celebrity buzz. Dr. Jones immediately goes out and starts marketing the surgery. He puts up PPC ads on Google that send people to his website, hoping he'll book some surgeries.

Unfortunately, Dr. Jones doesn't have any good before-and-after photos of his work. He also didn't bother to examine what the competitors are doing so he can position his services to be uniquely advantageous to his competitors.

Dr. Jones puts more and more money into marketing the service but the sales simply don't match what he's spending. Eventually, he decides the surgery is not worth it and abandons the effort prematurely. Dr. Jones scoffs at a fellow colleague, who seems to be advertising for the same surgery. He buys another ticket for the roller coaster and hopes for the best on the next ride.

However, his colleague, who we'll call Dr. Smith, thinks strategically. He has the same need to fill surgical time and has also spotted the opportunity. The first thing he does is call in his marketing consultant. They sit down and discuss how to best implement the available tactics toward the strategic goal.

The consultant identifies that Dr. Smith doesn't have enough before-and-after photos and tells him to apprentice in order to get some surgeries under his belt. He also notes that the competition is performing the augmentation with implants and there is a rising trend for fat grafting.

While Dr. Smith starts apprenticing and gathering photographic proof and new techniques, the consultant goes to work on differentiating the surgical offering. He positions both techniques and Dr. Smith as uniquely advantageous in comparison to Dr. Jones and the rest of the market.

The stage is now set. The landing pages are up, the educational materials are in place, and Dr. Smith has gathered the minimum of photographic proof required. His apprenticeship has also had an unexpected effect. He's beaming with confidence and ready to take on the world.

The strategy is in place and only now do they begin the offensive. The online ads go up and the search engine optimization efforts are on their way. The unique positioning also allows for a press release to go out.

The visitors that click on the ads are persuaded to take action and contact Dr. Smith for a consultation. The consultation was part of the strategic plan, so it converts well. Dr. Smith is soon busy with surgeries. He has no time to look at his marketing. Thankfully, his marketing consultant is busy at work optimizing the campaigns. He notices that print is not performing and shifts more of the attention online. The surgeries keep building. The tactical offensive is a success and the strategy is proven and justified.

Dr. Jones hears of Dr. Smith's success and all he can do is turn green with envy.

In my consulting experience, I see this scenario played out over and over. I watch doctors jump on the bandwagon and implement senseless tactics that don't perform. They then turn around and tell me that everything from online marketing to print ads simply doesn't work.

The key thing to understand about strategy is that if your objective is sound, and you know where you're going, you can afford to try multiple tactics until the strategy is a success. Implementing tactics without strategy is like walking around while wearing a blindfold. You could very well get to your intended destination, but you'll probably get hit by a bus instead.

Strategy is the overriding idea, the thirty-thousand-foot view of the situation. It allows for rational decision making and is the container that allows for fluidity in your tactical implementation.

So, What's a Business Plan?

Too often I see people confuse business plans with strategy. I largely look at business plans as a complete waste of time and the best way for you to limit your growth. Business plans lead to budgets; budgets lead to rigidity; and rigidity leads to loss.

In what feels like another life, I was sitting in an office with a young man who held a position a bit beyond his years. I was there on a temporary consulting basis to handle some matters requiring creative direction. It was December when the corporate collective stupidity decided it was time to fire people, set a budget, and then rehire people in January because they were short-staffed.

The young man began to tell me how impressed he was with his boss, who was able to set the budget in December and, nearly to the penny, stick to it by the end of the following year. He was in awe of her ability to predict the coming year's budget.

The only thing I was thinking was, "Wow. What a pathetic way to limit your growth potential." And that's exactly what that company did. They failed to innovate because they were too busy covering their corporate asses with planning. They made none of the changes I suggested, and about a year and a half after my consulting stint, they went out of business.

"Goal setting has traditionally been based on past performance. This practice has tended to perpetuate the sins of the past."
—Joseph M. Juran

Strategy vs. Planning

Strategy trumps planning every time. Strategy tells you where you need to be and then allows for the fluid implementation of tactics based on market conditions and market reaction to those tactics.

Planning says that you have to spend a certain amount on print advertising that year. Strategy says that you have to acquire a certain number of new clients. The available tactics include print, which is tested and then evaluated.

Planning says you need to spend X amount of money on PPC ads. Strategy tests your PPC campaign and determines the ROI. If the ROI is significantly advantageous, planning does nothing while strategy begins to pour as much money into it as is available and reaps massive growth.

Strategy has an unlimited growth potential. Planning can only grow within the confines of the plan.

Now, I'm not advocating that you should never plan ahead, far from it. I do, however, want you to make a clear distinction between a traditional business plan and strategic planning.

The rules to successful strategic planning are simple:

1. **Start with the end in mind.**

2. **Set a testing budget to determine ROI, but never set a fixed budget for any initiative.**

3. **Always check your tactical implementation along the way and adjust.**

4. **Once you hit on something that works, and you can prove it's scalable, pile as much money into it as possible.**

5. **Never do ANYTHING that doesn't work towards your strategic objective.**

There are two times when I see no alternative to a traditional business plan: when you're trying to get a loan from a bank or dealing with a narrow-minded investor. At those times, I suggest you hire yourself the best business-plan writer you can afford and don't waste your time on dealing with the plan. Spend your time on strategy and implementation.

WHERE STRATEGY FAILS

While discussing the difference between doing business in Canada and the US, my friend said, "With the Americans, you get either a *yes* or a *no*. With Canadians, you get a very definite *maybe*."

While I won't generalize, I found that very funny because it reminds me of where even the best strategic plans fail: implementation.

Five frogs are sitting on a log. Four decide to jump off. How many are left?

Five. Because there's a distinct difference between deciding and doing.

The number one failure in business is failure to take action. It's tempting to talk until you're blue in the face about what you should do and how great it's going to be. This kind of intellectual masturbation is rampant. The more intelligent the person the more they indulge in it. I've been guilty of it myself in the past because it feels great to flex my brain, to figure out how to do something. The mistake is in thinking that the work ends at figuring it out.

Implementing strategy is the single most important thing you can do in your business. The only difference between a loser and a winner is the degree of implementation. It's not enough to figure out how to run. You actually have to train for the race, and then run it. If you're a thinker, find yourself a doer. If you're a doer, find yourself a thinker. I've yet to meet many doctors that are brilliant at both strategy and implementation. The one or two I've met got too busy to implement and were stuck on the roller coaster. You need to identify your strengths and your weaknesses and then put the right people in place around you to help implement.

I want to stress this. **Implementation is the single biggest factor contributing to your success.** Even the best strategy will fall flat on its face if you don't implement it.

> *"He who has a why to live can bear almost any how."*
> —Friedrich Nietzsche

Learning to Fail

The single largest benefit of implementation is failing. That's right—failing is good.

You're probably trained to believe that failure is bad. During surgery, I'd have to agree. However, in business, you want to fail and fail quickly.

If you're not failing, you're not learning. That's the simple truth. Every time you fail, you get invaluable feedback from the market. You can then use that feedback to adjust your course. The keys to failing are to fail quickly, fail often, and fail strategically.

That's not to say that you can't learn from success. Success is great, but it's the fear of failure that stops you from reaching success. I've also noticed that success tends to drive people away from examining the situation because they're too busy enjoying the ride. When you get success, you don't need any prodding to go on and this can make you complacent. By definition, success rarely stops anyone from achieving their goals.

I'm not afraid of your success. I'm afraid that a fear of failure may stop you from TRYING. So let's talk about failing and why it's so great.

FAIL QUICKLY

When you're implementing a new marketing idea, it does you no good to wait for months to find out what works. In the days of print advertising, we used to have to wait for weeks to find out what worked and what didn't. In today's world of online advertising, tracking, and testing, you can get feedback within minutes of your ad going live.

Never implement any new initiative without conducting at least some testing online. With online ads, you can very quickly test how the market will react to a new visual, a new phrase, or new idea. If you're thinking of optimizing your site for a new key term or service, don't do it until you've first tested the market with some safe PPC ads. Why buy a piece of equipment on the say-so of the manufacturer? Put up an ad and see how much interest there is for the new machine in your area.

The quicker you get feedback, the quicker you can adjust your course. Think of it as putting one of those old windup toys in an empty room. It hits the wall and changes course. It does this a few times and eventually finds its way to the open door. The faster you wind it, the sooner it will succeed. Failure is good. Learn to embrace it as the doorway to success.

> *"Success is the ability to go from failure to failure without losing your enthusiasm."*
> **—Sir Winston Churchill**

FAIL OFTEN

Now that you understand the need to fail, you need to not only do it quickly but also often. Testing should become a habit. It should happen on a daily and weekly basis in your practice. Everything from the greeting you use on the phone to the way you close a consult should be tested. The more often you try things, the more intelligence you'll collect. The more intelligence you have, the stronger your strategy will be and the more effective your tactics.

FAIL STRATEGICALLY

Failure for failure's sake is not the goal. Remember that you should never implement anything unless it furthers your strategic goal. When you set yourself up for failure, it should be for a specific reason.

- **Don't run ads unless you're trying to get data at the same time as you try to get business.**

- Don't change your phone greeting unless you're tracking it and seeing which converts better.

- Don't implement any test unless you need specific data to make a change.

When you start with the end in mind and you know where you're going, failure is just part of the process. No degree of planning will ever replace solid feedback from real-world experience. Failing strategically means failing for a purpose. Define your purpose, define the objective, and start implementing.

"I've missed more than nine thousand shots in my career.
I've lost almost three hundred games.
Twenty-six times, I've been trusted to take the
game-winning shot and missed. I've failed over and over
and over again in my life. And that is why I succeed."
—Michael Jordan

CHAPTER 8

Is It an Expense or an Investment?

Investing in your business marketing is the single biggest financial leverage you can have.

It's easy to look at your marketing as an expense. It costs money like anything else. But your marketing should never be an expense. It should always be measured and looked at as a profit centre. It's the single best investment you can make.

The largest fortunes in the world were made on the backs of businesses. Bill Gates didn't get his wealth by putting his money in the stock market or letting some unqualified financial advisor tell him what to do with it. He built his fortune by building a business, and countless others have done the same.

When you devise strategic, measured, and innovative marketing, you increase your upside potential to virtually unlimited heights. You can control your investment and decide how big or how fast you grow.

The narrow-minded doctor will look at marketing as a cost.

He'll try to cut corners and pay the least amount possible. He'll usually attract mediocre results from mediocre companies and he'll be pleased with his ability to save money. Unfortunately, he'll completely miss the purpose of his practice. It's not to SAVE money. The purpose of any enterprise is to MAKE money.

There is nothing wrong with watching your expenses. It's important to know what you're paying for and that you get value. But never make the mistake of confusing an expense with an investment. An expense has no yield. An investment returns money on your payment.

If your marketing can return a multiple of what you invest, it's in your best interest to invest as much capital as possible in that marketing.

Marketing in a Down Economy

When times are tough, the temptation is to cut down on your expenditures. It's very tempting to look at your marketing spend and think that it needs to be reduced. This is a critical error made by many practices. Once you reduce your marketing, you reduce your income. Your patient flow suffers and your cash flow is eliminated.

What typically follows is a series of further cuts followed by the inevitable staff layoffs. Good people are let go and service suffers soon after that. The net result is a diminutive business, incapable of servicing clients and a mere shadow of its former self.

The moment you start cutting your marketing, your practice starts to die. I've seen this over and over. The businesses that manage to survive through tough economic times are never able to get back to their former glory.

So What Should You Do When the Economy Is Not Behaving?

If you're suffering in a down economy, it's because you're not properly differentiated and have poorly performing marketing. All our clients have seen tremendous growth in the middle of a global recession. We've never had a company falter and not grow. At the time of this writing, the cosmetic industry is in the midst of a downturn. Our clients are thriving and operating at full capacity.

The reality is that people still buy even when the economy is sputtering. Even if 50 percent of the market vanishes, that still means that 50 percent of those customers are still buying.

When tough times hit, the first thing your competitors do is cut their advertising expense. Their strategic error is a huge opportunity to steal market share. As they contract, you should expand. You should take up any space they forsake and put more into your advertising and marketing. By being more aggressive during a downturn, you position yourself to emerge from it with a much larger market share.

Even if the market drops, your business can grow by scooping up more of what's left. You can double or triple your business in a down economy and come out of a recession as the dominant player in your market simply by out-advertising, out-marketing, and out-maneuvering your competition. You'll learn to love a recession and how it shirks off the players that were simply riding the wave of good times. You'll take market share and dominate as the largest player in the market using the business you won from all the other doctors that pulled back to "save" money.

CHAPTER 9

Marketing Not Only Attracts But Also Selects a Customer

I often get asked about whether ramping up online marketing will lead to a flood of tire kickers and looky-loos. That's certainly a possibility if your marketing is not positioned well and if you leave your patient encounters up to chance.

The job of your marketing shouldn't simply be to attract a patient. It needs to control that patient's perception of you and allow you to have firm, yet benevolent, control of the relationship.

For example, if you're the kind of doctor that makes himself available to all new patients by phone and email, that sends both positive and negative messages. It can say that you're friendly, caring, and available. It can also say that you're a loser that has lots of free time and nothing else better to do. Successful people are not available. People want to deal with successful doctors. They don't want your personal email and phone number. They're silently pleading to be lead and guided. There are ways to make a patient feel comfortable and cared for without becoming their whipping boy.

You can also use your marketing process and the Buying Roadmap to vet your prospective clients. For example, there is often a big debate about charging for a consultation or offering it for free. Both have advantages and disadvantages. If you charge, you're certainly going to stop some people from coming to your office. If you publicize that on your site, you'll reduce that interest even further. What you will also do is remove the vast majority of tire kickers and increase the quality of your surgical consultations.

If you offer a free consultation and your positioning matches, you can expect to see a lot more people, but more of them could be of lower quality or located very early along their buying journey.

For me, the decision to charge or not to charge largely boils down to how I position you. If you're a young doctor without a lot of surgeries booked, I'd advise a free consultation. It will fill your waiting room with patients and make good use of your downtime. I'd then focus all the attention on the in-office conversion process to turn as many of those potential tire kickers into buyers. As you get busy and your money-generating activities increase, you can strategically switch to a paid-consultation model.

The important thing is not if you charge or don't charge. What matters is that you charge and don't charge at the right time and for the right reasons, based on a strategic direction that supports the growth and continued expansion of your practice as well as your desired quality of life.

When your marketing process is properly vetting, selecting, and aligning your patients with your strategic goals, you can spend more time doing the things that make you more money and that you love to do. Every decision in your practice should drive progress towards the overall strategic vision for the practice and your personal aspirations for your definition of success, be it money, family, or fame, and in whatever mix of those elements suits you.

Should We Continue the Conversation?

You've come to the final chapter of this book and are excited—ready to apply the Practice Growth Formula to your business. You can see the potential in your practice, and you now know how to realize it with the Formula. Hopefully, you're excited about the possibilities and are starting to feel a sense of control and optimism over your ability to attract new and better patients.

This book has detailed the unique psychology of the plastic surgery buyer and the persuasive voice that communicates to her desires. I have demonstrated that **activity does not equal progress,** and how doing what *you* do best and allowing others to do what *they* do best is the key to your exponential growth—coupled with a positioning and differentiation of yourself, and your procedures, so that you're recognized by the buyer as the best in your field, for them. You learned vital information on how to convert your leads into patients, fulfilling every need along the Buying Roadmap and avoiding fatal strategic and tactical marketing mistakes.

You can certainly apply all that you've learned to achieve the growth and success that you deserve, as we have done for our clients. But is that the best use of your time? Is it an 'A'-level activity, as you learned in Chapter 3? It's usually not, and that's where we come in.

At Think Basis, we apply the Practice Growth Formula to help our clients saturate their consultation schedule and convert more prospects into paying patients. Most doctors worry about filling the waiting room and avoiding the tire kickers. For our clients, the situation is the opposite. People are put on long waiting lists and pay for their surgery ahead of time just to secure the date they want before another patient snatches it away. Our clients don't chase after patients or waste time with a lot of tire kickers and bargain hunters. Our marketing does all the selling for them, well before a patient ever sits in front of their desk. It ensures a high degree of quality consultations with qualified patients who want our clients as their surgeon (and not a random surgeon that will knock off an additional 5 percent).

We pride ourselves on providing a hassle-free experience. We'll never ask you to write content, update your Facebook page, or, heaven forbid, "tweet." We take care of your online needs and keep your website updated and converting well without you having to provide pages and pages of text. That doesn't mean you'll be excluded or not have final say on the materials produced in your name—quite the contrary. We welcome your oversight and, at least in the beginning, we'll ask you to approve all the content so we can learn your style and comfort level. The only work you'll have to do is assign a liaison from your office who provides photography, makes sure that content and press releases are approved in a timely fashion, and keeps our web team current with in-practice events, promotions, and developments.

More important than the online activity, you'll spend quality time with an expert on positioning and uncover the core of what makes you unique, special, and advantageous. The process will uncover traits of your business that we'll use online to win market share. You'll then use these traits in your practice and for your consultations to boost the overall conversion rate, translating it into higher profits and increased satisfaction. Being in business will become fun again. Nothing tastes as good as winning, and we have a strong taste for victory when it comes to the cosmetic surgery business.

On top of the physical work performed, you get the assurance and security that comes from being aligned with a company that's a hundred percent focused on knowing what works online and how that fits with the trends in cosmetic buying. You'll never again have to be alone and unsure about your marketing. You'll be tapped into an expert source of information that's being constantly battle-tested in the real world for effectiveness and profitability.

I don't, however, want you to think that this will be all play and no work at the office. You're going to have more consultations and more surgeries than you've probably ever had at any one time in the past. You'll be talking a lot and cutting a lot. Until you grow to a level that justifies bringing on junior surgeons and expansion, there is no way around that. The difference is that you'll now be working on the activities that actually **make you money,** as opposed to the fruitless Facebooking, tweeting, and web updating of the past.

Before you read on, I should tell you about the kinds of clients we don't work with. We typically can't take you on if you're completely new to the industry and have no experience, proof of your work, or the financial ability to sustain the effort for at least six months without stressing out about it, while we work to transform your positioning, your marketing, and business. While we're good at what we do, we can't perform miracles and things don't happen overnight; they take time. We also can't work with you if you deliver poor-quality work, reflected in numerous online reviews and a poor industry reputation. We can only take on reputable surgeons with a track record of quality and accountability for their work.

The other times we've run into issues, has been with surgeons that have a hard time letting go and trusting in our expertise. If you're addicted to doing things yourself and think that nobody can do anything right unless you have your hand in it, we won't be working together for long. Even though our clients stay with us for years, we do routinely fire clients, and refuse to contract with surgeons that are not a good fit for the reasons stated above.

If you're a quality surgeon with a solid portfolio of before-and-after images, and you're ready to take your practice to the next level and meet or exceed your past personal, professional, or financial goals, let's continue the conversation.

We have a simple pricing structure that starts at just $10,000 per month. This fee increases over time based on meeting performance and profit objectives, but caps out at $15,000 per month.

If you get just three to four additional surgeries a month, our services are paid for in full. If you take the lifetime value of that client into consideration (the amount of money she's likely to spend with you on BOTOX®, creams, laser, and other treatments), your investment returns a long-term profit even at the very conservative figure of three surgeries a month.

In addition to our fees, you're responsible for all third-party spend, such as Google pay-per-click advertising, printing, and other technology costs, such as email systems or software. Our fees do include hosting and other costs associated with the maintenance and performance of your website.

I use the term *investment* very deliberately because we should not be seen as a cost centre to your business. Our Practice Growth Formula creates a marketing machine that drives business to your practice every day of the week. Compare that with print advertising that can cost as much as $12,000 and only appears for a single day, and you see that there is no comparison.

There is one more thing. Because we work with clients on an area-exclusive basis, we can take on only one surgeon per area. This means that if one of your local competitors beats you to it, you're out of luck and we can't take you on until that client either leaves or we fire him. We could put you on a waiting list, but the period we work with clients is usually measured in years, not months.

At the end of the day, if you're not willing to invest in yourself, why should your patients invest in you? Was that too harsh? It wasn't meant to be. It's just the reality of the situation.

The next step is to schedule what we call a "discovery meeting" where we have a relaxed thirty-minute discussion and mutually evaluate if, and hopefully agree that, we're a fit for each other. You'll be asked to provide your current website for assessment ahead of the meeting, as well as possibly any supporting material that allows us to confirm your ethics and quality of work if it's not easily identifiable through our online vetting process.

Please contact Andy Edur at Think Basis at 647-557-6085, or write to him at andy.e@thinkbasis.com to arrange for your free meeting. We look forward to working with you and making your success a reality. Imagine not having to worry about where to find, and how to convert, new patients.

Whether you implement the formula yourself, or let us do it for you, do something!

Bibliography

1. (Botulinum Toxin. Retrieved from http://en.wikipedia.org/wiki/Botulinum_toxin.)
2. (Buyer's Remorse. Retrieved from http://en.wikipedia.org/wiki/Buyer%27s_remorse.)
3. (Kingmaker. Retrieved from http://en.wikipedia.org/wiki/Kingmaker.)
4. (Strategy. Retrieved from http://en.wikipedia.org/wiki/Strategy.)
5. (Tactic. Retrieved from http://en.wikipedia.org/wiki/Tactic.)

For more information
please contact Nick Dumitru's office at
info@thinkbasis.com

CPSIA information can be obtained at www.ICGtesting.com
Printed in the USA
LVOW10s1111201213

366213LV00002B/47/P